MW01255073

ROUN

FACING THE ABDOMINABLE

Memoir of a Young Colon Cancer Survivor

LISA FEBRE

Black Rose Writing | Texas

ISBN: 978-1-68513-266-8
PUBLISHED BY BLACK ROSE WRITING
www.blackrosewriting.com

Printed in the United States of America
Suggested Retail Price (SRP) $22.95

Round the Twist: Facing the Abdominable is printed in Minion Pro

*As a planet-friendly publisher, Black Rose Writing does its best to eliminate unnecessary waste to reduce paper usage and energy costs, while never compromising the reading experience. As a result, the final word count vs. page count may not meet common expectations.

To Louis, my Crow.
May your wounds heal, too.

PRAISE FOR
ROUND THE TWIST:
FACING THE ABDOMINABLE

"A deeply personal, honest and informative account of one young cancer survivor's journey, her prose is easy on the eye and mind; her stunning comparisons of the good and bad in nature are intelligently woven throughout, and her inspirational soul emanates from every page, as if she hasn't already given enough. Able to make you weep one moment and then guffaw the next, Lisa's book is a beautifully written testament to the power of love, friendship and self-worth, and is essential reading for cancer sufferers, cancer survivors or the cancer curious."
–Neil Baker, Author, Owner April Moon Books

"If you are facing a life-threatening illness or any kind of hardship, you should read *Round the Twist: Facing the Abdominable*, by Lisa Febre, a remarkable survivor of colon cancer. In Febre's detailed, raw, honest, humorous, and mesmerizing story about battling and surviving both cancer and the ensuing treatment, you will be inspired by what can be accomplished through courage, tenacity, spirituality, and hope. This is a must read."
–David B. Seaburn, PhD, Assistant Professor, Psychiatry and Family Medicine, University of Rochester Medical Center (retired), and author of nine novels, most recently, *Give Me Shelter*

"*Round The Twist* is a memoir about being incredibly alive and deeply loved. Lisa Febre's journey through the best and worst of what modern medicine has to offer is crackling with detail, intensity, and wit. A balm for the soul, a love story in disguise."
–Emily Wright, Assistant Editor, *Strings Magazine*

"Statistics don't lie most of us will be or will know someone diagnosed with cancer, but *Round The Twist: Facing The Abdominable* by Lisa Febre is a book that explains the author's cancer journey with insight, humor, forethought and empathy for not only other cancer patients, but those who love and care for them. Lisa's journey is not for the faint of heart, but one that honestly and openly chronicles her cancer diagnosis, treatments and life-changing experience. She lays her soul bare at a sometimes-heartbreaking level while readers are left understanding the fight so many of us face when the word cancer comes out of our doctor's mouth. This book will open the reader's eyes to the battle that is cancer survival and shine a spotlight on Lisa's strength and courage while giving others hope that there is light at the end of battle."

–Barbara A. Luker, author of *The Right One*

"Lisa tells her story with so much heart, such candor, one is drawn into her narrative right from the get-go. I laughed — yes, laughed. I cried. With her easy-going prose, Lisa welcomes you along on her harrowing journey — with the sole purpose of helping others understand what it is like to endure all the tests, all the treatments, all the ups and downs of fighting cancer. For those facing "The Big 'C'", for those who know someone enduring the unimaginable, *Round the Twist* is must-read."

–Melinda Wolf, Writer and Editor

"*Round the Twist: Facing the Abdominable* submerges you into the dark reality of a Stage-4 Cancer diagnosis where survival is the only option. An inspiring, emotional investment sending the eye-opening and powerful message that even when a diagnosis is dire, miraculous healing and restoration can happen with a top-notch medical team at your side and allies who feed your mind, body, and spirit in tandem. Truly inspiring!"

–Michelle A. Dick, Freelance Writer, Editor

ROUND THE TWIST:

FACING THE ABDOMINABLE

"Gone 'round the twist" is slang that implies someone has gone crazy. Certainly, with my cancer diagnosis, my life went 'round the twist. The visual of going down the U-bend in a pipe appealed to me as an allusion to the sigmoid colon (the body's U-bend) and to describe this whole crazy experience with colon cancer.

This story is my version of the events that transpired after my diagnosis, pieced together from my sketchy memory, peppered with stories my husband told me of events of which I have no memory, and the many journal entries I wrote during this period of my life. I have changed a few of the names for privacy and moved some events around in time for narrative purposes, but everything included in this story happened.

PROLOGUE

5:30 on the morning of my final chemotherapy infusion, my dogs discovered and chased a rabbit around our backyard. They were unrelenting in their pursuit, all three animals racing to either escape or inflict death.

After securing the dogs in the house, I found the little rabbit lying flat on the ground next to our ancient olive tree. Carefully, I picked her up in my hands, feeling her racing heart, pumping lungs, and unimaginably soft fur. She lay unmoving in my hand. I gently turned her over and felt all the parts of her body, searching for signs of broken limbs or bite wounds. She seemed to have come through her ordeal unscathed. I returned her to a hole in the fence and she hopped away into the dark safety of our neighbor's dogless yard.

This event has stuck with me as the perfect metaphor for my brush with cancer.

Like the rabbit running for her life, I, too, would drive myself to the edge of death trying to escape colon cancer. Whatever amount of energy I had to sacrifice to fight this thing, I would give. No matter what terrain lay in my way, I would not stop until the danger was gone or until the chase killed me.

For over a year, I was engaged in the ultimate run for my life. In December 2021, I received a diagnosis of Malignant Neoplasm of the Sigmoid Colon, Stage-IVC[1]. In the 10 months that followed, I endured 4 surgeries, 12 weeks of chemotherapy, and 29 rounds of radiation. I suffered through all the physical side effects, emotional traumas, painful recoveries, and sleepless nights one would expect during cancer treatments. Against all odds, I escaped the chasing monster. And I would do it all over again if it meant I can remain here on Earth for just a little longer.

I was determined that cancer would not take me down. No matter what I faced, it would not change who I am, and I would not let it consume my head. Cancer will always be a part of me, stalking from the shadows like a dog sniffing for hidden rabbits in the garden. How long I can stay hidden remains to be seen. But I know one thing for certain: I need to be even better at hiding than I was at running.

Cancer is not a disease that is *cured* in the conventional sense. Chemotherapy, immunotherapy, radiation, surgery, and all the modern medical interventions may kill, zap, attack, and remove it from my body, but cancer will never be gone from my life. I can fight it and I can do everything in my power to outrun it, but it will always be a specter haunting my trail. Living out the rest of my life with the shadow of cancer on the edge of my periphery, I will continue to be tested, poked, prodded, scoped, bled dry, cut into, or scanned. Cancer may be forever, but I refuse to live in a perpetual state of fear and uncertainty.

I find myself another rabbit in the garden, hiding from cancer and recovering from this near-death experience, exhausted from running for my life.

---

[1] pT4a pN2a pM1c For more information on cancer staging: https://www.cancer.org/cancer/colon-rectal-cancer/detection-diagnosis-staging/staged.html

PART ONE

"This is all temporary." — *Dr. Edwin L Jacobs*

I, Lisa

Against the empty whiteness of the computer screen, the cursor blinked at me with persistent expectation. The rhythm mesmerized me, the symbolism paralyzing. My husband had suggested that I write about my cancer treatments in real time to help me sort through the very complicated emotions I was experiencing. It sounded like a great idea until that January afternoon when I sat down, intending to follow his advice. Filling the blank page with words seemed impossible. So, despite how ridiculous it seemed, I took a deep breath, set my fingers on the keyboard, and typed, "Once upon a time, there was a little girl named Lisa." The first hurdle cleared, this wild horse was off and running.

I never imagined myself as a writer. My focus had always been on music. But I have been typing for almost as long as I have been playing the piano. My mother gave me her old Smith-Corona manual typewriter when I was 8 years old. It came in a groovy, dark green, hard shell carrying case which I had to store under my bed. I could barely lift it, it felt like it weighed more than I did. Every time I popped open the buckles, the familiar combination of dust, oil, and ink hit my nose. I can still smell it as if it were right in front of me. My mother taught me how to touch type on that old beast.

Typing as fast as I could think, the world of imagination opened for me. No longer limited to the stories that other people wrote, I was making up my own. I would sit on my bedroom floor and type for hours on end. The sound of that old manual typewriter echoes in my memories. Even as I typed these words on my silent computer screen, I could still hear the nostalgic click-clack-ding-slide.

In high school, I wrote a few articles in the school newspaper about the music and drama departments. My teachers encouraged me to write *Letters to the Editor* of our town newspaper, and at some point, my English teacher told me to consider pursuing critical writing in college. None of that fit into my life plan. While pursuing my music degree, I still found time to enroll in a few writing courses and continued to write for my edification.

After college, writing became a hobby. My focus was on my fledgling music career, but I enjoyed writing creative monthly updates to my music students and started a food blog back in the *olden days* when food blogs were a novel concept. In recent years, I was a regular contributor to a vegan magazine, and now I write the monthly newsletters for a local orchestra. I have always been told that my writing style is accessible and honest, and people seem to enjoy reading whatever it is I write. With both pride and terror, I accept that compliment.

I understand I lack formal writing training and a polished technique since I just write what I hear in my head. Regardless of the subject or what format I was using, I saw I could use writing to reach a broader audience. So, when I began blogging about my cancer journey and discovered that close to 1500 people in at least four countries were following along, most of them strangers, I embraced the revelation that my writing was helping people. Maybe I could bring comfort and illumination to those who found themselves overwhelmed by their experience. Maybe just one cancer survivor would discover that they are not alone inside their heads. Perhaps I could help someone find hope within the darkness of cancer. If my story could touch just one survivor or patient, then this effort was all for something.

I love being in the spotlight. I have been a musician since I was 4 years old. The world is my stage. No matter where I go, I am convinced that all eyes are on me. My husband, Louis, has said that if I were a cartoon character, I would pop through every door, arms outstretched, announcing my arrival with my very own catchphrase: "Ta-Dah!" Despite my outward ease, confidence, and charm in almost any social situation, it might surprise people to learn that I have phone anxiety. I am desperate to find excuses to cancel social engagements, and I am likely to push away new friends the moment it seems we are getting close.

As a child, animals fascinated me, and I spent hours learning everything I could about them. From the chipmunks and squirrels in my backyard to the exotic creatures I read about in the *National Geographic® Books for Young Explorers* like elephants and dolphins, I felt affection for all animals. And above all, I was crazy about horses. To this day, my love of animals is an overriding character trait that directs my actions at all turns. I have stopped on busy roads to pick up cats hit by cars, carried baby birds back to their nests, and have eaten no meat since I was 16 years old.

Overall, I had an unremarkable childhood. I think that makes me pretty darn lucky. My younger brother Todd and I had a happy, normal, stable childhood in a Levittown-style neighborhood in Rochester, NY. We grew up in a little house with a small backyard, with parents who were, and still are, happily married, and all with a cherry on top: a white cat named Snowball. We took a summer-long cross-country family road trip when we were teenagers, which resulted in some excellent family inside jokes. We still laugh about my behavior during an infamous stop at the Crater in Arizona and my brother panning for gold in Colorado at a roadside tourist trap, with the intense belief he was going to strike it rich. Our parents carted us to swim meets, hockey and football games, band concerts, music lessons, babysitting, and landscaping jobs without complaint. We learned to drive a stick in our father's pickup truck, and how to balance a checkbook at the kitchen table. We enjoyed the adoration and attention of our parents and because of this, we both thrived with the confidence to pursue our chosen passions. No matter what path we took, we knew there was always a safety net, our parents holding a big round striped trampoline, frantically shadowing us to catch us in case we fell.

While in college, majoring in music, I met my first husband. We got married one year after graduation, our enthusiasm blinding us to the obvious fact that we were way too immature for any of this adult stuff at that age. Inevitably, as we grew up, we would grow apart, which had already happened by the time we purchased our first house two years into the ill-fated marriage.

The little Victorian home, built in the 1850s, stood in North Adams, a cozy little town tucked away in the Berkshire Mountains of Western Massachusetts. I loved every moment of those five years we lived in that house. Like me, it was small but mighty. When our young marriage was struggling, we had home improvement projects to keep us distracted from the real problems. When I was home alone every weekend with the new baby, an actual ghost in the attic kept me company.

During the scariest moments of chemotherapy, dark hallways formed in my brain that terrified me to explore. To calm my nerves while I lay in bed listening to the chemo pump, I would imagine walking detailed tours of that old house. I would enter through the tiny mudroom and step into the modest kitchen; my small music room was next, separated from the living room by a squeaky pocket door. The youthful version of my beloved cat, Dusty, sprawled out on the radiator in the dining room, would muster the minimal effort required to raise his head and watch me walk past. Next, onward to the staircase built with 14 steps because, in the 19th century, 13 steps were unlucky. I remember the third step from the top had a creak that we tried but could never fix. Our son Andrew's nursery was at the top of the stairs, painted sky blue with white clouds, which *Pop* of the mom-and-pop paint store down the street, taught me to do with a sponge. The first door on the left, the guest room, had walls which I had daringly painted a deep berry color that profoundly worried my mother. ("What if you change your mind?" she fretted upon seeing it for the first time. "I won't!" I promised, and I was right; we moved out long before I would ever repaint). The long hallway had no more doors until the end: a tiny bathroom, which had once been an actual water closet. The last door was to a little room with a secret connecting door through the closet to the master bedroom. My memory tour would end with me standing at the foot of the old bed, a view of Mount Greylock out the window.

I would return to reality to find myself more at ease with what was happening to me. The pump next to me in the bed was not as ominous; the drugs were not as scary.

I was more in love with the house than with the husband. Then again, given how things turned out between us, I am not surprised one bit. The best thing to come out of our troubled 12-year marriage was our son, Andrew. All along, we were good friends, but that was never enough. So much was missing. I wanted love.

Soon after our divorce in 2009, I met my second husband, Louis, in what would be a continuing whirlwind romance. We met by sheer chance and dumb luck. Introduced on a whim by a mutual acquaintance, I marvel at the unlikelihood of our meeting: I grew up in New York; he grew up in Mexico. Thirty-Five years later we met in Los Angeles, hugging like old friends who had not seen each other in a while. My heart still skips a beat when he walks into the room, no matter how much time has passed since that first meeting. We both had a second chance at genuine love, and we grabbed onto it with both hands. I always expected to feel this way about the person I married, like I exist only because they do. We were married in 2011, and all these years later, I love him more.

Unfortunately for my mother, Louis is a composer. She had once dreamed that I would become a doctor. Obviously, I did no such thing. In two marriages, I did not even marry one. The lifestyle of musicians can be hard for others to understand. Louis likes to describe it as *living in the space between the trapeze swings.* It can look stressful from the outside, but musicians get it. It is all part of the fun.

Louis is 15 years older than me, which is not a big deal. Though, I get a little sad knowing I will probably spend the last years of my life alone. Fate has guaranteed me to watch the love of my life leave this world. We had always talked about that future, so we planned and saved for my security after him. Of course, we never considered that it might be me who checked out first.

He has encouraged me to take flying leaps of faith in my career. For 20 years, I was a professional oboist, cultivating a solid and gratifying career. During a concert, I suffered a unique injury that would take that all away. At an unexpected crossroads, I had a choice: feel sorry for myself and give up or go forth and try something new. For me, the choice was obvious. I would try something new. With my husband's support, I stepped onto a fresh path, working to forge a new career as a cellist. Louis never pushed me to settle into a more comfortable place. He supplied me with all the tools I needed to take on this exciting new challenge. I think he was pretty brave to do that for me. This was one of the greatest gifts he ever gave me.

In the fall of 2021, we were still settling into our new house, making plans for redecorating. We moved in three years ago. Yet the living room still held a mishmash of items from our old place, making us look like a couple of college grads in our first apartment with hand-me-down furniture from our parents' basements. We were collecting supplies for a backpacking trip to Catalina Island that we were hoping to take the following summer, and happily going about our everyday business.

That is when cruel fate decided it was time to smack this pony on the ass.

• • • • •

In the summer of 2021, the COVID pandemic was running into its second year. By now, the lockdown measures were slowly being relaxed. The world was opening up again for normal activities, like indoor dining at restaurants. I only cared that we musicians got to perform again. The orchestras that I belonged to were giving careful and safe outdoor summer concerts, just to dip our toes back into the pool after 18 months of silence. During my first post-lockdown concert in July, I felt the first twinges of the pain that would come to be diagnosed as a symptom of colon cancer.

At 47, I am old enough to know I am not invincible. A few high school and college friends have died, so I know that life is short. I can still take a few risks now and again while understanding that I am not 30 anymore. Enough of my daring friends have broken collarbones in bicycle crashes for me to know we do not bounce off the pavement. I know the value of owning a home, having a nest egg and a retirement fund, and that taking a vacation now and then is important to maintaining my sanity and my marriage. Not yet contemplating my mortality, old age still seems far enough into the future that it is unfathomable to see myself at 80. At this age, my body is still strong and viable. I have very few grey hairs, so I still get carded by flirtatious servers now and then.

Cancer is supposed to happen to other people. Cancer is something that happens to strangers and characters in a movie. It was so far outside my safe and comfortable reality that I never stopped to consider for one second that the weird pains I felt might be a symptom of something serious. It must be a little constipation or menstrual cramps. Why would I jump to the conclusion that it was cancer? I am perfectly healthy. I take no prescriptions for anything. I am vegan[2] and I exercise daily. The last time I had a physical, my doctor gave me a clean bill of health. *I don't need to worry. Take some Advil, go to the bathroom, and get back to work.*

---

[2] https://health.clevelandclinic.org/the-best-diet-to-lower-your-colon-cancer-risk-2/

Based on the statistics, no one is exempt from cancer. Even if you are not the one diagnosed with some form of it, someone you know will be. Thanks to my diagnosis, every single person I know now knows one person with cancer. These days, it feels unavoidable. The best we can do is learn from others' experience, so on the off chance we are the person with cancer, we might have a few extra tools with which to help ourselves cope.

Being a young cancer survivor, by which I mean I am under 50, comes with a lot of strange feelings. I feel I am entitled to a deep sense of accomplishment, having just witnessed the incredible feats my body was capable of, though always tempered by a sense of sadness. Cancer has taken something from me. I can feel the hollow space it carved into my heart, even if I am not sure what used to be there. Often overcome with waves of grief, I find myself face to face with the childhood memory of a grey pony, crying over a lost dream I can never get back.

While I drifted in and out of morphine dreams, I saw Louis weep inconsolably; as we have laid together on our bed, I have felt waves of anxiety pouring off of him; and I have looked at my 21-year-old son, who lost his father when he was 10 years old, and realized he was terrified of losing his last remaining parent, but doing his best to hold his shit together for my benefit. I do not know if either of them thought I was actually dying. For the first time, we had to face the reality that any of us could be gone in the blink of an eye — our spouse, our parent, ourselves.

I find amazing beauty in the scraggy grass in our backyard, the barking of the squirrels, the circling hawks, and the way the wind moves through the trees. I have cried while listening to Beethoven and Debussy. I have hugged my body; I have thanked it for what it did for me. And I have accepted that there will be a time when the two of us will have to part ways.

In August 2022, eight months after my diagnosis, five months after I completed chemotherapy, and one month after radiation ended, I held the results of a third PET scan in my hands. Numb and in disbelief, it was difficult to accept what I was reading on the page. I carried the papers around with me for a week until they were wrinkled and creased, expecting words to materialize out of a puff of magic smoke which would confirm something terrible. Maybe I needed to un-focus my eyes to make the 3D image of a deadly cancer cell appear or use an invisible-ink-revealing pen to see the buried secret message. I could not allow myself to believe what I saw with my own eyes was true; it felt like some sort of spell had been cast, fooling the PET machine into not detecting any new hypermetabolic activity in my body, missing the spots on my liver claiming they were nowhere to be seen, and pretending that by all appearances I was a perfectly healthy human.

That night, as we lay in bed, tears came pouring out of me. I cried as if my life depended on it. A flood of emotions gushed from me in waves of sobs and tears. Some were familiar old friends; others were nameless feelings I have never known before. I cried on and off for about an hour while Louis held me and wiped my cheeks during each new torrent. At some point the storms calmed and I fell asleep.

When I awoke the next day, a beautiful world stretched out before me. "Hooray, hooray, a brand-new day!" I cheered with my exuberant dogs, who are always happy and enthusiastic every morning. They never seem to wake up on the wrong side of the bed. I want to be like them: full of wonder and amazement just because the sun came up. The thing I mourn now is not my mortality, but that it took this brush with death to appreciate the simple act of waking up.

THE GREY PONY

When I was a child, my parents had friends who had a hobby farm, complete with a retired thoroughbred and a very sweet, old, grey pony. We would visit them every summer, and I would spend most of my time at the barn, petting the horses. Their daughter, with whom I was supposed to be friends just because we were the same age, made the visits very unpleasant. When not tormenting her little sister and my brother, I was the target toward which she satiated her appetite for cruelty. She would lock me in the basement and turn off the lights while all our parents were upstairs playing cards after dinner and oblivious to the drama playing out below their chairs. Once, she led me into the woods behind their property and then ran off, leaving me to make my way back alone. I dreaded our summer visits to their farm but loved getting to sit with the horses.

During one such visit, when we were about 10 years old, and knowing how obsessed I was with her horses, she tempted me with a ride on the old, grey pony. I was beside myself! All the parents gave their permission, so we went out to the barn alone. She showed me how to brush the quiet little pony before putting on the saddle.

She gave me a leg up, and I was on. I held the reins, and the pony walked quietly around the riding ring with me glowing on his back with contentment. My heart bursting with the thrill of pure, innocent happiness in the way we only feel it as children. This extraordinary moment remains one of the most joy-filled memories of my childhood.

And then it happened. I heard her mirthless laughter just before she smacked the pony on the rear end. The little horse bucked and ran as fast as he could. I hung on to the reins for dear life as the world streaked by in bouncing tunnel vision. When the wild ride ended, he stopped at the far end of the corral and stood quietly as if nothing had happened. I untangled my fingers from his mane, slithered down from the saddle and cried, pressing my face against his and hugging his neck. She yanked the reins roughly from me. Dragging the obedient pony back to the barn, she roared with laughter and relentlessly teased me about being a scared little baby.

I was crying because she had hit the horse. To deeply understand who I am, you need to know that story.

FACING THE ABDOMINABLE

According to the National Institute of Health (NIH), 39.2% of Americans will have some type of cancer in their lifetime[3]. In cancer math, that works out to roughly two in every five people. For context, I played with a quintet in college: five random, unrelated musicians. One of our members, Jeremy, was diagnosed with non-Hodgkin's lymphoma in 2018, so statistically speaking, one more of us would meet the same fate.

That someone was me.

In 2021, people were supposed to get their first colonoscopy when they turned 50. Being that I was 47 and at a (seemingly) low risk for colon cancer in particular, it appeared safe to allow me to wait those three years before having the test. Nationwide, though, colorectal cancer cases were on the rise in people under 50[4]. The American Cancer Society would not announce the new screening age of 45 until mid-2022, several months after my diagnosis. Usually, I love to be on the cutting edge of new trends, but this is one I wish I had avoided.

[3] National Institute of Health, National Cancer Institute. Bethesda, MD, https://seer.cancer.gov/statfacts/html/all.html
[4] American Cancer Society https://www.cancer.org/latest-news/colorectal-cancer-rates-rise-in-younger-adults.html

It was incredible the speed with which life went from unremarkable to absolute bananas. I can count the months, six of them, from when I became concerned about a mysterious pain to when I received my diagnosis. It began as a low simmer, sending up the occasional little bubble of doubt and fear, the frequency increasing with accelerating speed until we hit the boiling point in December 2021.

For some people, a cancer diagnosis might play out the way they often portray it on television: a dramatic scene where our protagonist has an acute attack of pain, violently coughs up blood, then passes out on their kitchen floor; the character's doctor takes immediate action to scan and test them in a slick montage of the most high-tech hospital machines and futuristic facilities imaginable; followed by a bright whitewashed scene in an austere mahogany-trimmed office, sitting across from a stony-faced, well-manicured oncologist with his hands folded on his desk who says in a cold monotone voice, "You have cancer," everyone breaking down in hysterical tears. "Why me, why?" It all happens in three minutes of filmmaking.

None of this happened to me. It took a couple of months for me to worry about the pain and even longer before I googled *symptoms of gynecological cancers* and *symptoms of colon cancer*. Once I was seeing the correct doctors, they were already volleying around the possibility of cancer like they were tempering eggs. My diagnosis did not come out of the blue. In the words of Chandler Bing, it was "smack dab in the middle of the blue." I was sober. I did not even shed a tear when the doctor confirmed it was colon cancer. Everyone had given me plenty of time to get used to the idea. Finally hearing the official diagnosis, my only reaction was, "Now, what do we do?"

Not all doctors assume their younger patients (by younger, I mean anyone not considered geriatric) have a low tolerance for pain. I am not claiming that many still subscribe to the antiquated notion of hysterical women. But it seems like too many of them shrug us off without digging deeper. A woman I have known since elementary school might have been saved if they had taken her complaints of back pain seriously from the start — she suffered for nearly a year before her cancer diagnosis, and by then it was too late for her. As my story played out, it was crystal clear which doctors took me seriously and which ones were more than willing to look past my complaints to see what they wanted to see. The first set of doctors only wanted to look for cancers that fit their area of expertise and were not seeing the whole person. It almost cost me my life, too.

All I needed was for someone to hear me.

Family history is, of course, a huge part of the pirate treasure map that guides our doctors to the giant X hidden somewhere inside of us. My father has had two types of cancer in each of his kidneys: in one, papillary urothelial carcinoma, and in the other, transitional cell cancer. He will most likely receive immunotherapy for the rest of his life. Neither of my father's diagnoses seemed to alarm any of my own doctors. Because these cancers were most likely caused by environmental factors, my brother and I were at low risk. He is the closest relative I have who has had cancer. My father had three uncles who had colon cancer. The assumption was my great-uncles were too far removed from me to be of any genetic interest. Doctors were always more focused on my mother's sister, Lorraine (breast cancer), and my mother's father (prostate cancer).

Overall, I had a very low risk for breast cancer, but that did not stop me from having my yearly mammograms. My whole adult life, my physicians reassured me that my history of endometriosis did not increase my likelihood of developing any gynecological cancers. Regardless, I still had yearly ultrasounds.

Everyone seemed perfectly content to continue along this path of annual screenings and physicals. Receiving the confirmation that I was in excellent general health became routine.

Of course, there is always the possibility of a gene mutation causing a cancer which is unrelated to known family history. When unexpected cancer pops up, they may do genetic testing to uncover an underlying genetic risk factor that no one knew about. The unfortunate luck of unknowingly buying a house in a nuclear waste zone could trigger a mutation in our DNA. At this point in human history, I believe it can be nearly impossible to live somewhere that is free from any sort of chemical or radiation pollution. Moving to the South Pole to live off the grid is unrealistic. We must figure out how to survive in this contaminated world we have inherited.

My father and I are very similar in both our physical fitness and general lifestyle. Neither one of us has ever smoked. We eat healthy diets. We both exercise daily and have done so for our entire adult lives. And of course, for the first 18 years of my life, we lived in the same place — a place teeming with industrial pollution. It was, therefore, likely that his family carries a genetic predisposition toward certain mutations that could lead to the cancers we both have, triggered by our exposure to varying levels of radiation and chemical pollution throughout our lives.

With my diagnosis, several doctors asked me if there was a history of Lynch Syndrome in our family and if we were of Ashkenazy descent. Although my father's family immigrated from that region of Eastern Europe, I had no answer to those questions, and neither did my father. We both underwent genetic testing. But at that point, what did it even matter? We both had cancer. We already knew the punchline.

At this point in my story, I was not interested in picking apart the reason I had cancer. I was more interested in surviving it.

•   •   •   •   •

I became expert at twisting and deforming the facts of my case, no matter how plain they were to see. Before going through this serious illness, I could never imagine how virtuosic I would become at this. During the months leading up to my diagnosis, I was guilty of some incredible mental contortions that would make any circus performer envious. It is important that I be honest as I explore and expose the process I went through to accept my diagnosis, certain that I am not the only person who has reacted like this. Just about everyone out there struggles to come to terms with their new cancer diagnosis. The struggle made harder if they do not present with textbook symptoms of a specific cancer.

At 28, and after a long diagnostic process, I found out I had endometriosis. Beginning with my very first period, I experienced intense cramping. My doctor accused me of having low pain tolerance — just take more Motrin. When I was 23, I started passing blood with bowel movements. Without a full exam, my doctor told me I had hemorrhoids, and I needed to eat more vegetables. I had been a vegetarian since I was 16; how many more vegetables did I need to eat to cure hemorrhoids? Even my gynecologist thought little of my painful cramps. To them, I was probably just another hysterical young woman, and they had patients with more pressing maladies to deal with.

It never felt like anyone took my complaints seriously, so I continued on with no relief from my symptoms. During the first trimester of my pregnancy with Andrew, I began experiencing terrible cramping. I was terrified and stressed, convinced I was going to have a miscarriage. Over the next few months, the pain diminished to a more tolerable level and the rest of my pregnancy progressed without incident. And just to prove to everyone that I did not have a supposed low pain tolerance, I gave birth with no drugs. After Andrew was born, I breastfed him, which held my periods and the accompanying pain at bay for over a year.

On New Year's Eve, when Andrew was 14 months old and just beginning to wean, I experienced intense pelvic pain and was rushed to the ER. Eight hours and a parade of doctors later, we were no closer to finding the answer to what was causing the pain. Specialists ruled every gastrointestinal issue out until finally one general surgeon (to whose daughter, incidentally, I was giving piano lessons) listened to me and theorized that I had ovarian cysts. She ordered an immediate CT scan, confirming her suspicion: multiple ovarian cysts had formed on both ovaries; the largest, the size of a lemon. She believed that the pain was from one or more cysts bursting.

The next year would mean a lot of tests to diagnose the greater condition. I was placed on hormone therapy to control the cysts, which meant I had to speed up Andrew's weaning. The return of my periods brought more intense pain. For the next year, I had monthly ultrasounds to track the growth of new cysts, a memorable MRI during a blizzard at a hospital two hours away, the process culminating in laparoscopic surgery to remove multiple ovarian cysts, the largest measuring 6.4cm (about the size of a tennis ball). During the surgery, the surgeon discovered my pelvis and all its contents to be a sticky mess. Endometrial lesions were on virtually every single organ, including my bladder and colon. She removed as many lesions as she could while saving my ovaries. I was 29 and Andrew was

2 years old, too soon to know if I wanted more children. She worked hard to save my ovaries, leaving the option for more babies; and unbeknownst to her, she also left me the ability to save my life from colon cancer two decades later — the ovaries were the canaries in the coal mine.

After surgery, they gave me a drug called Lupron for six months. I never had that theoretical second child, so I was on continuous hormones to control the endometriosis for the next 20 years. It appears to have worked because when the surgeon removed the cancerous portion of my colon in 2021, he said that I showed no signs of endometriosis. No one seemed to want to laugh when I said from my hospital bed, "Thank goodness it's not endometriosis, it's just cancer!"

In June 2021, a week after receiving both doses of the COVID vaccine, I began a 22-day menstrual period. It may have started out as just a coincidence, but 22 days is not normal bleeding for anyone except women who have just given birth. During this period, I had intense cramping, which did not stop when the bleeding stopped. I put up with these abnormal lingering cramps for a couple of days, then I called my gynecologist.

I love my gynecologist, Dr. Silberstein. Similar in age to me, we also jog in the same park where we sometimes spot each other. I trust her completely. She brought me into the office for an exam and ultrasound within days of my distress call. She reassured me that the period was just an unfortunate coincidence with the vaccine. It was the ovaries that concerned her the most: a cyst the size of an orange had formed on the right one and she could not get a clear picture of the left one through my colon. The pain I was feeling was probably from that 7.6cm cyst, and another of similar size on the hidden left ovary. She would need to repeat the ultrasound in four weeks to track my progress. Women with ovarian cysts know that this is how it goes: watch and wait. I had been through this so many times, over the past two decades, that I knew the drill by heart.

When I returned for my follow-up, the right ovarian cyst was shrinking. Still, though, my colon obscured my left ovary, meaning she could not get a clear picture of it. The pain on that side was increasing, and so was her concern. Dr. Silberstein was uncomfortable waiting four more weeks for another in-office ultrasound, advising me to call my primary physician if the pain got worse or new symptoms popped up in the meantime. Her suspicion was that the pain was coming from my colon, not the ovary.

For a few more weeks, the pain was intermittent and did not raise any red flags. But then it began interfering with my ability to work. The start of the concert season is a busy time for musicians, and I had several concerts lined up. Although I was not experiencing what anyone would call severe pain at that point, I noticed it was becoming uncomfortable to sit in my seat for an entire three-hour rehearsal. When I moved around during breaks, I would get some relief. I powered through the first three concerts, so I convinced myself that I had a handle on the whole thing. I could go many days in between bouts of acute pain, and it was not all that severe. Yet.

In October, I had even more concerts booked. I found that keeping busy provided a mild distraction from the growing pain. Fighting my way through all the rehearsals and performances, I was barely holding myself together. The other cellists noticed I was losing weight and not acting like my usual energetic self. Mid-month, I backed out of a concert two days before the performance, something I have never, ever done in the three decades of my career. Two weeks earlier, I played a concert which I thought I had managed well; but the pain had worsened so quickly that neither sitting nor standing was comfortable.

A new pain, deep in my pelvis, appeared. A dull ache in my lower back joined in. I had difficulty urinating, and my bladder was full to bursting. My primary physician cautiously diagnosed a mild urinary tract infection and immediately started me on antibiotics. I had no relief. The pain in my pelvis persisted, the antibiotics were not working, and the back pain was getting worse by the day.

All women know that there is a big difference between gynecological pain and everything else. I knew something was wrong. I knew it was not gynecological. But the scary stuff, like cancer, had not even crossed my mind.

I was in so much pain I was giving up many of my normal activities. I had stopped trail running; I avoided taking the dogs out for walks, their brisk pace was too much for me. Even though I had an appetite, if I ate a sizable meal, I would get intense intestinal pain soon after. Practicing yoga was the only thing that gave me some relief. I had lost seven pounds in three weeks. I can do food math: I know that eating fewer calories leads to weight loss, but it did not compute that I had a raging appetite yet continued to lose weight.

My brother arrived in Los Angeles for a short three-day visit. I struggled to keep my shit together. Todd is not blind; he saw that something was wrong. We went out to dinner one evening and, because I was always starving, I ate an enormous bowl of risotto. I was awake all that night, with terrible, unproductive intestinal spasms. These were not cramps. They were spasms. I groaned with every bowel movement. It was awful. The next morning, Todd and I went on a long hike. While we were out on the mountain, I told him about everything. Hearing myself describe the situation out loud, I realized this was more serious than I had wanted to believe. He was rightfully worried about me, and I reassured him I would call my doctor the next day after we dropped him off at the airport. I was worried, too.

What I had not told him, or Louis, was that at night, when I laid on my back in bed, I could feel a long lump growing in my belly near my left hip bone and that when I pushed on it, it hurt. This was the same thing that hurt whenever I tried to use the bathroom. By now, I had severe constipation. It was obviously *not* my left ovary.

It was time to stop pretending this all would just go away. I had a real problem. Something was going terribly wrong inside me. I had two choices: give in to the fear and become paralyzed or do something about it.

•　　•　　•　　•　　•

My primary physician is a brilliant man named Dr. Lee Kagan. A talented diagnostician, he is infinitely curious about the world. He loves to share his knowledge of anatomy and medicine and fill his listeners with as much information as they can stand to absorb. I have had some interesting conversations with him during my physicals because it is also clear he recognizes when someone else is curious about whatever topic is being discussed. Incidentally, we discovered he was a resident at Highland Hospital (Rochester, NY) the same year I was born there. It is hard to dismiss the wonders of the Universe knowing, as a young doctor, he was nearby when I was born; 47 years later, in a city across the continent, he saved my life.

Dr. Kagan is the sort of doctor who I never feel embarrassed to talk with about any topic to do with my body; he is one of the few doctors who truly listens to my concerns. I had no reason to feel anxious about having to discuss my pooping habits with him. And yet there I was, in my car, rehearsing the exact words I would use to open the conversation about my bowel spasms and constipation. It was going to be of critical importance that I did not play coy; I needed to lay everything out there as plainly as possible, so there was no mistaking my level of concern. I knew I would not be leaving his office with a diagnosis of irritable bowel syndrome (IBS) and a new meal plan. This was serious business, and I gathered up my energy, focusing it to prepare for accepting bad news with grace.

"I think there's something wrong. I have a pain here" — I pointed to the left side of my pelvis — "and I'm having a lot of pain with every bowel movement." Obviously, I had nothing to worry about. He grabbed the reins and began directing the conversation along the correct roads. Immediately made clear through his eyes over his surgical mask, this was not ovarian cysts or a sensitive stomach. He was genuinely concerned. It looked like I would need mountains of courage to face what came next.

Other colon cancer survivors have asked me what symptoms I had that drove me to see my doctor. I only had two of the classic symptoms of colon cancer: constipation with persistent pain. Unexplained weight loss, overall, is a symptom of just about every type of cancer. When I saw Dr. Kagan at the end of October, I had lost 7 pounds, just enough to raise some eyebrows. Over the next six weeks leading up to my surgery, though, my weight spiraled down 16 pounds, which is a big deal for a woman of my small stature.

The symptoms I did not have were diarrhea, bloody stools, weakness, and fatigue. Turns out I was very lucky to have had so much pain (if one can call themselves lucky for pain), because it forced me to seek medical care sooner rather than later. I have heard too many stories from other survivors, saying they had no symptoms, or that their symptoms mimicked food poisoning, and so they dismissed them. Most times, it was a coincidence that the doctors discovered their colon cancer at all.

I met Suzy while we were both having chemotherapy. Just a couple of years younger than me, she had shown none of the symptoms of colon cancer. She had no clue that something was going wrong inside of her body. Just happened that one day she felt a strange lump in her neck and called her doctor. After seeing a few specialists, they concluded that cancer had metastasized throughout her body and caused the swollen lymph node in her neck. It took more tests and scans to figure out it was colon cancer. I cannot imagine the number of sleepless nights filled with *what ifs* she had; how long could she have gone with no symptoms?

Although I had only two symptoms to work with, Dr. Kagan's mind was made up: this was not IBS. Something serious was going on and I would need a CT scan. *Stat.*

On November 1, 2021, exactly one week after that appointment, I was sitting in another waiting room, drinking contrast dye, and preparing for a CT scan. Being sick in the Age of COVID was a very lonely business. Not allowed to bring Louis in with me, I sat in the waiting room fretting in solitude. I was shaky, nauseous, and on the verge of tears. Despite the flurry of texts we exchanged, I was utterly alone to manage my fears.

They led me back to the changing room area, where lockers line the walls and anxious people in flimsy hospital gowns sit in cold, uncomfortable chairs awaiting their turn in some giant machine. A little boy, about 4 years old, with a broken arm and dressed in a pint-sized hospital gown, was clinging to his mother. I broke my arm around that same age, and I remember how frightened I was at every doctor's appointment. The broken bone had been so painful. I was always worried that someone would do something to my arm to make it hurt again. He was probably expecting more pain awaiting him through the metal door with no windows.

The technician began pulling hospital gowns from the shelves and instructed me to remove my jeans and anything with metal. "For the abdominal scan."

The little boy's eyes widened and flew up to my face. He tugged anxiously at his mother's sleeve. "What's an Abdominable?" His panic rising, his wide eyes never leaving me. He probably expected me to transform, like a werewolf, into some nightmarish monster right before his eyes.

His mother reflexively shushed him. His first lesson in how to censor himself instead of using honesty in the face of medical care. I smiled wide enough so that he could see it in my eyes above my mask, and I patted my belly for him. He looked relieved that a fantastic beast would not jump out and devour him. I felt better, too.

Little did he know, he had coined the term that I would use to describe the Monster growing inside of me: *The Abdominable.*

As I climbed up on the table, there was no way to predict what this CT scan might reveal. I had not yet allowed myself to freak out about the scarier possibilities. At the very least, I knew it would show some ovarian cysts. But beyond that, I could not imagine. All I kept thinking about was if our new insurance company would cover the bulk of this bill. Feeling guilty for spending money so close to the holidays, I was dreading more tests and procedures that would cost us even more. I vowed to look up our deductible when I got home so I could start moving money around, expecting a tsunami of bills surrounding all these tests.

One thing I definitely was not expecting was for Dr. Kagan to call two hours after I got home. The instant his name popped up on my phone screen, my heart leaped into my throat, and I felt a sick green panic rising. For a brief second, I considered not answering. Is a diagnosis real if no one is there on the other end of the phone to hear it? Of course, I answered. As he spoke to me, I could feel myself losing grip of just about everything, his words coming at me like they were being piped over the old public address system at school, distorted and distant, yet urgent and authoritative. I wanted to cry; I wanted to laugh; I wanted to get off the phone.

Louis watched me from across the room, unable to hear the doctor's voice. But I could tell by his face that what was coming through the phone into my ear was bad news. Dr. Kagan said something about a gynecological oncologist, then told me he would call the next day after he spoke with Dr. Silberstein. "Don't panic. We don't know anything yet." During the call, I had walked across the room in a trance. I found myself standing over Louis, who was sitting on the edge of his favorite chair.

"It isn't good," I heard my voice tinny and distant. I was numb and calm. "There's a 10cm cyst on my left ovary, with a 3cm solid mass inside it. He's not sure what that is, but he wants to send me to a gynecological oncologist." Tears leaked from my eyes, but I was not crying. All the parts of my body forgot how to work together: my mouth spoke the words, but I felt like a remote observer; my legs were weak, yet my brain refused to let me sit down.

I have great difficulty trying to remember what happened over the next week. This stretch of time is cloudy, each of these memories floating around my brain as vignettes without time or context. I remember calling my parents while sitting in my yoga-slash-music room to tell them what was going on. The moment the word *oncologist* passed my lips, my father let out a horrible sound that I never want to hear him make again. Of course, this sent me into hysterical tears. Speaking to both of my doctors at various points, their familiar voices bringing me back to earth as they advised me to take it one test and one appointment at a time. A stack of vials of blood was drawn, leaving me with bruises on the inside of both of my elbows. I made the appointment for a PET scan while riding in our car. I have no memory of Dr. Kagan giving me the order for the PET scan; and why I made the appointment from the car is even more of a mystery.

All of this is a blur.

My train was about to jump the track. Our instinct was to accept the oncologist referred by Dr. Kagan. Louis has been his patient for almost 30 years, I have been with him for 12, and in all those years, he has always sent us to great specialists. We should have followed his advice this time, too. Instead, we went with another oncologist who we found through our insurance database. I had all the right reasons for going to this one first. Assuming this was ovarian cancer, the insurance company could not deny any treatment claims for a doctor on their own list. It was all very reasonable and lucid, and so we moved forward.

One week to the day after my CT scan, we were sitting in Dr. Messina's office[5], preparing to hear what we knew would be bad news. Dr. Kagan did not send me to an oncologist because he thought it would be a fun way for me to spend an afternoon.

---

[5] Although Dr. Messina is a real doctor, the name has been changed

He sent me there for a damn good reason. Yet I tried desperately to convince myself this would all turn out to be for nothing.

After a rough pelvic exam, Dr. Messina said, "Did anyone talk to you about your liver?"

Louis and I looked wide-eyed at each other, completely blindsided. "No?" I was still lying on my back with the thin paper sheet over my knees.

Snapping off the exam gloves like a character on *Grey's Anatomy*, Dr. Messina casually walked to the door. "Get dressed and we'll discuss it when I get back."

Our stress levels were rising like teapots. I felt ill, and I could see that Louis was bubbling with anger. It was heartless to make a declaration like that, walk out the door, and make us wait to hear the explanation.

Upon returning, Dr. Messina performed a dramatic reading of my CT scan. This Emmy-worthy monologue was accompanied by an elaborate sketch of the body with all the questionable spots that appeared on the scan emphasized. I felt we were being patronized. Louis and I are not dumb-dumb stupids. We know what a uterus looks like and, with 20 years of experience, I am pretty good at reading ultrasounds and recognizing blood-filled endometrial cysts versus fluid-filled follicular cysts. I know what a liver looks like. Little arrows with the names of organs on them are unnecessary. I was annoyed long before the doctor began the explanation of what the scan showed.

Yes, yes, we know: a 10cm cyst on my left ovary, with a 3cm solid mass encapsulated within. *I know what an ovarian cyst looks like. No need to draw one. Ok, never mind. Just tell me: when are you taking that thing out?* There was some question about something the radiologist had referred to in the report as *thickening* of the sigmoid colon. Since Dr. Messina was not a colorectal surgeon, I was absolutely not interested in any musings.

What was the most off-putting was the air of vindication. Dr. Messina was the brilliant scientist who discovered the spots on my liver first and was planting a flag. Apparently, there were three lesions that showed up on the CT scan. According to Dr. Messina, this was the absolute indicator of metastatic cancer. "But from where? That little 3cm ovarian mass?" How was it possible that I would go from no cancer a couple of months ago to metastatic ovarian cancer? I had no symptoms of ovarian cancer. Why was Dr. Messina spit balling, live and on air, with the patient? We would have to wait for the PET scan (scheduled for the following week) to know exactly what we were dealing with. In the meantime, I would get a referral to an actual colorectal surgeon to see what was going on in my colon.

We left the office with more questions than when we had arrived. Spots on my liver? Does that mean I have liver cancer or some invisible aggressive cancer that the CT scan is not showing which has metastasized? Could a 3cm ovarian tumor be the source of three metastases in my liver? None of my pelvic lymph nodes were swollen, nor did any show up on the scan. In fact, no lymph nodes anywhere in my body would light up on the upcoming PET either. Maybe I just have some sort of autoimmune disease which causes liver damage, and those are not cancerous lesions. What does any of this even mean? Does anyone know what the fuck is happening inside of me?

I spent the next week in sheer panic.

Ahead of my PET scan, we met with the colorectal surgeon. Dr. Unger[6] initially made a good impression as likable, pleasant, thoughtful, intelligent, and having a firm command of the

[6] Although Dr. Unger is a real doctor, the name has been changed

subject of large intestines. After going over my medical history and the CT scan results, it was time for a rectal exam. No big deal. I was expecting this, as every doctor seemed to want to poke and prod every one of my orifices for the past two weeks. I was used to it by now.

I did not see the sigmoidoscopy coming, though. The doctor explained that it might be uncomfortable because of the air that needed to be injected into the intestine for the scope to have space to move around. *Uncomfortable* is hardly the word I would choose to describe a rigid sigmoidoscopy. It was simply medieval torture, comparable to having a tooth drilled without Novocain.

My poor little colon, which had already been giving me daily pain, was now screaming in agony. Louis looked terrified. My head checked out for a few minutes because my memory of this whole episode is foggy. I would later find out that not only is the rigid sigmoidoscopy[7] rarely done anymore, but it is also supposed to be done under sedation. *Who's got a low pain tolerance now, Dr. Hemorrhoids?*

"Ah yes, there's a tumor." Dr. Unger spoke from somewhere around my butt region. There must be a better way to tell a patient you see a tumor than while there is a camera up their ass. With the scope extracted, Dr. Unger prepared the supplies for a biopsy. I was completely defeated. How could I endure this physical and mental pain a second time? I lay unmoving on the exam table, fighting waves of panic and fear. All the while, a little voice inside my head chanted "… a tumor… a tumor… a tumor…"

Dr. Unger reinserted the scope, and the sharp pains and spasms returned instantly. After what felt like an hour-long

---

[7] https://my.clevelandclinic.org/health/treatments/10749-proctoscopy-rigid-sigmoidoscopy

struggle to get the biopsy[8], he claimed to have gotten a small sample. He would send it out right away. I could expect to have the results in a couple of days. In the meantime, we went over how surgery to remove a cancerous stretch of the colon would work: the surgeon removes enough colon to get clean margins (which means leaving only healthy tissue behind, no cancerous cells), along with the adjoining lymph nodes. We were told that this surgery is very common, colon cancer is very common, and many people go on to live long and productive lives.

Although it sounded like scary news on the surface, hearing the casual description of the surgery gave me a lot of comfort. Ok, if this turns out to be cancer, we just cut it out and I go on with my life? Is this really the worst news possible? From what I have heard, ovarian cancer is much scarier to treat and harder to survive. I should be thankful that no one is talking about that mass on my ovary anymore, right?

I left the exam room feeling positive, convinced that I would just have surgery and then, like magic, I would be cured. Chemotherapy or radiation or any sort of treatment beyond this was unthinkable. I believed I would be just that lucky.

The nurses at the front desk told me that the doctor would call with the biopsy results, and they would schedule the colonoscopy for later that week. We would also need to talk after the PET results were in. I felt confident that things would happen fast. It seemed reasonable to expect that in just a few days, I would have some concrete answers. I left feeling a little more optimistic than I had in days.

After the elevator doors closed and we were finally alone, Louis said, "He had a hole in his sock."

---

[8] There was never a tumor *inside* my colon, which was why there was a "struggle" to get a biopsy

Wednesday, November 17, 2021: PET scan. Unlike Dr. Kagan, neither Dr. Messina nor Dr. Unger called me that same afternoon to relay bad news. Instead, we heard nothing from either of them for several days. I tried to convince myself that *no news is good news,* but no matter what I did, I could not bring myself to actually believe it. I wanted to call Dr. Unger's office before the weekend, so on Friday, I attempted to do just that. The nurse who answered the phone told me they had not yet received the PET results from the radiologist, nor the biopsy results from the pathologist, but I should call back Monday (11/22) to schedule a colonoscopy.

An appointment with Dr. Messina scheduled for the upcoming Wednesday (11/24) led me to assume I would get the PET results then. Instead, what we were told at that appointment was scattered and confusing. According to my negative CA-125 test results, I did not have ovarian cancer. Dr. Messina's attitude after that confirmation was one of "my work here is done, move along," and mild annoyance when we continued to ask questions about the rest of the scan. The PET showed the same inflammation in the sigmoid colon. Again, the radiologist commented it was probably not cancer because of the size of the affected area. Of the three lesions on my liver, only one showed hypermetabolic activity, meaning that one was a metastasis of some cancer. Then Dr. Messina declared I would have to start chemotherapy right away.

I was confused. *Do I or do I not have cancer?* In the beginning, I may have been resistant to finding cancer, but now I worried that while these doctors were blowing me off, some deadly cancer was growing unchecked inside of me. I no longer trusted Dr. Messina. No way would I let this person tell me I needed chemotherapy. No one even knows what kind of cancer we might be talking about. I could not accept the wishy-washy explanations, so I certainly would not accept the deadly serious prescription without a concrete diagnosis.

We could not get out of that office fast enough. As we drove away, we agreed we were never going back.

In the meantime, my multiple calls to Dr. Unger's office continued to go unanswered. The nurse would reassure me each morning the doctor would call me back that afternoon. I never received a single call. This was unforgivable. A doctor should never say to someone "You probably have cancer" and then blow off their calls for a week. I understood that Thanksgiving may have caused a slight delay in the speed with which the office returned calls, but this was more than that. I was being ignored.

My friend Ella had the most rational assessment of the situation. "Remember, a gynecological oncologist is looking for gynecological cancers; a colorectal surgeon is looking for colon cancer." She was right. No one was looking at the *whole Lisa*. Just bits and pieces. It was confusing and stressful and unproductive.

Frustrated, I called Dr. Kagan and asked if we could come in to have him read the CT and PET scans. We needed a lucid voice in all this chaos, someone we trusted to give us straight information without an ulterior motive and who could deliver what we now expected to be bad news with compassion.

Meanwhile, the pain that I was experiencing was becoming unbearable. I used to think giving birth was the worst pain I had ever felt. My sensors had to be recalibrated because this intestinal pain was off the charts. I spent every night writhing in our bed, holding a heating pad on my abdomen, and taking Advil with Tylenol, which now did nothing for the pain. I was reaching the end of my rope; the pain was affecting my ability to think straight. Louis wondered out loud every night, "Is it time to go to the emergency room?"

The following Monday morning (November 29), we finally felt like we could breathe again. Dr. Kagan sat at his desk, reading over the radiology reports to himself *before* addressing us. He took in the information first and did not just read it back to us like the other doctors had been doing. He knew we had been feeling overwhelmed and lost for the past two weeks. We appreciated this.

He confirmed what we were suspecting on our own: all signs pointed toward colon cancer.

"How could I go from being perfectly healthy to suddenly having colon cancer? How could this happen?" I asked him.

"You did nothing wrong to make this happen." He was doing his best to reassure me, but I still felt I had somehow failed. He read my mind as simply as he had read the scans. "There's no justice in this world," he added. Although the news was scary, he kept telling me that this is one of the most common cancers, that the treatments can be very successful, and that within his practice, other patients had beaten colon cancer and, years later, are living normal and healthy lives. This was the second time I heard this, but coming from Dr. Kagan, I gave myself permission to believe it.

His first order of business was to get our derailed train back on track, and the only oncologist to whom he felt he could entrust my care was Dr. Edwin Jacobs (PMI Oncology at the Disney Family Cancer Center, Burbank, CA). Before the week was over, Dr. Kagan would contact him himself to line up my care. My heart skipped a beat at this news: not only was a grownup finally in control of the situation, but my father's oncologist is also named *Dr. Jacobs*. This had to be a sign. I was going to be ok.

He would also attempt to get the biopsy results from Dr. Unger, so he had his assistant call the office. She returned a few minutes later to confirm the phone number because the response she received from that office was, "We have no record of a Lisa Febre here."

Up to this point, I had been slowly slipping over the edge, struggling to hold myself together. But this was too much. I burst out in near hysteria, tears streaming down my face. "He stuck a scope up my ass. I definitely remember him!" She went back to her desk to call the office again. I imagine whatever she said to them in the next phone call was not as polite as her first attempt because when she returned this time, she had information. They had received the biopsy results, which came back inconclusive. They claimed they had not scheduled a colonoscopy yet because there was a problem with my insurance. I found it difficult to believe, much less trust, this message.

Dr. Kagan gave me explicit instructions: call Dr. Unger's office every day at 9:30 a.m. and again at 2:30 p.m. until I got Dr. Unger himself on the phone. If I did not speak to the doctor by Friday morning, I was to report back to Dr. Kagan. For the next three days, I did exactly as he instructed. Every time the desk nurse answered the phone, she told me the same thing: "Dr. Unger will return your call this afternoon, or tomorrow." No surprise. It never happened.

By Thursday afternoon, I had had enough. The final call sealed the deal for me. "Dr. Unger wants to do another sigmoidoscopy in the office tomorrow morning since we can't get you scheduled at the hospital for the colonoscopy." Something snapped in my head. I erupted in tears and, in a dramatic break from character, yelled into the phone: "No! I'm not going through another one of those things! I'm going to find another doctor!" I was astonished. The doctor had already told me I *probably have cancer*. How much longer was he going to make me wait? Anger coursed through my veins, easily overtaking my fear.

Some people have to hire a medical advocate to help them navigate the healthcare system; Dr. Kagan was mine. He took the wheel from this point on, scheduling an appointment on my behalf with another Gastroenterology Specialist. Pulling whatever strings it was he had at his disposal, he made the appointment for a colonoscopy consultation for Monday morning. He told me to expect fast movement from here on out. He predicted that I would have a colonoscopy within the week. Then, the new team of doctors would create a plan for the next steps. I was relieved, knowing he expected a diagnosis and treatment to begin soon.

Dr. Kashar's Physician Assistant saw me in the office the following Monday, and it was apparent to her that my situation was serious. To her credit, she was calm, poised, and professional when addressing my concerns. She palpated my abdomen and gave no outward signs of how serious this was. She saved me from being frightened by making sure that she had all her information before she told me anything. I appreciated her demeanor and ability to keep me calm. My sigmoid colon had swelled up so much in the last two weeks since the PET scan, it was now visible through the skin when I stood up. By this point, it was difficult to wear jeans or anything with a rigid waistband.

"Have you eaten anything today?" was her first question when she finished her exam. I shook my head no. Turns out, they were going to schedule my colonoscopy for the next morning. Finally, someone was doing something. No more guessing. No more runaround. My relief was intense.

For the first time in weeks, I could take a deep breath. But this would be the last one I would be able to take for the next year.

THE TWIST

I am pretty sure that I am the only person in the history of colonoscopies to enjoy the bowel cleanse the night before. For me, it was the first relief I had felt in weeks. Constipation had become so serious, despite two weeks of daily laxatives, that I had produced a *real* hemorrhoid this time, and the colon spasms were so painful I cried during every visit to the bathroom.

I showed up for the colonoscopy Tuesday morning, starving and nervous. Sitting in the waiting room, another patient noticed me staring hungrily at a ketchup commercial on the tv above our heads. "I'm hungry too," he said. I brightened at his observation and laughed.

"I could drink an entire bottle of ketchup and eat a pile of French fries and whatever that was in that last commercial, too!" This got the entire waiting room exchanging plans about what food we were going to indulge in once we got home. For just a few minutes, we all forgot how crappy it was to prep for a colonoscopy.

I had not met Dr. Kashar at the consultation the day before. We had to go through all the introductions in the procedure room. I was being pumped full of sedatives and not wearing my glasses, and of course, he was wearing his surgical mask, so I guess technically I still do not know what he looks like. "Dr. Kagan said you were a special case." He patted my arm. "I'm going to take good care of you." The pleasant drugs washed over me.

I had the kind of sedatives that did not knock me out completely. The drugs rendered me very much disinterested in everything going on, including the giant scope being stuck up my butt. I could see the screen, showing a lot of pink tissue, and I could hear what they were saying; although it sounded like a lot of gibberish, and I did not care. These drugs were great. I had forgotten what it felt like to feel no pain. I now understand how some people become addicts.

Louis had a sense of urgency about him as we walked back to the car an hour later. Thankfully, he did not break the news to me while we were walking, I am certain I would have collapsed in the parking garage. The tissue of my sigmoid colon had almost swelled shut, preventing the colonoscope from passing through. This time, the doctor got a real biopsy. Before I woke up, Dr. Kashar had already called Dr. Kagan with the report of the blockage. Dr. Kagan then called the surgeon, Dr. Philippe Quilici (Minimally Invasive and Oncologic Surgeon, Providence Saint Joseph Medical Center, Burbank CA) to make sure he saw me immediately and made an appointment for me for the next day. All I had to do was stay on a liquid diet for the rest of the day, not eat or drink after midnight, and show up on time to Dr. Quilici's office. I did not put together that these instructions were hinting at surgery the next day.

A blockage. As hard as I had tried to rationalize all my problems away as being related to endometriosis, a giant ovarian cyst, or an autoimmune disorder, a colon blockage was for real, and could be deadly serious. Obviously, there are many problems with something like this, mainly the possibility of my colon rupturing and bathing my entire abdomen in poisonous bacteria. Something very serious was causing the swelling. Unfortunately, the clock had already been ticking for months.

This was all exceptionally scary news. But I no longer felt fear. I felt taken care of. I felt at peace. It was because of Dr. Kagan's quick and confident actions that I was now getting the care I had so desperately needed. The Team of Grownups had been assembled and were in control. All I had to do was trust them. My head was clear, and I was ready for whatever was coming next. I would have freaked out if I had known just how fast the next part was going to happen, though.

Wednesday, December 8, I showered and dressed as usual. I gave Andrew instructions about what he should do with the dogs while we were at the surgeon's appointment. I grabbed my purse and told him we would be home for lunch. And that was all the preparation I went through before my surgery.

Dr. Quilici entered the exam room, personable, well-manicured, with a French accent decorating a deep baritone voice that did not quite match up with his slight frame. A man in command of his world. I counted myself lucky to be swept under his expert wings. After shaking my hand, he looked at me with warm sympathy. When he spoke, though, exasperation and indignation colored his booming voice and betrayed his cool exterior. "Who looked at your scans and didn't take immediate action?" In other words, *whose ass do I need to kick after school?*

"Do you want names?" I dangled the carrot. I caught a flash of intrigue in his eyes. Wisely, he declined with a twinkle. I was chuffed. We were going to get along great.

He palpated my swollen abdomen and then decided that fast action was the only answer. "I will help you," he said as plainly as if I had asked him to reach a book off the top shelf. At that, I burst out crying. All the weeks of fear, pain, uncertainty, distrust, and distaste came gushing out of me. I grabbed onto his arm, partly to steady myself, but partly to make sure this man who would surely save my life was real. "Thank you, thank you, thank you…" I chanted through the tears. He held my arm in his free hand and squeezed it with warm intensity. "You don't need to thank me."

I was now caught in a whirlwind. I was told to go across the street to St. Joseph's Hospital Emergency Room and tell them at the desk that Dr. Quilici was expecting me there. By being admitted as an emergency, I would not have to wait weeks for our insurance to approve the surgery. I was overwhelmed, confused, and struggling to grasp the severity of what was happening. I thought for sure I would have a couple of days to plan, pack, and prepare. I had not even refilled the dogs' prescriptions.

The ER nurse recognized that I was confused. She explained that I was going to be admitted to the hospital right away, and that I was having surgery the following day. She brought Louis back to visit with me in triage. He also tried to explain that I would not be going home. I was not grasping this idea. He hastily made a list of things he would get during a quick trip back to the house. (I still did not understand why I needed overnight supplies.) We lived over a half an hour away, so I would be alone to finish up the admission process. He kissed me for good luck. I went through the battery of pre-op tests and paperwork while he was gone.

Shortly after Louis left, a familiar face appeared from behind my bed curtain: Dr. Kagan! He stayed with me for about 20 minutes, talking me through what was about to happen while he did my pre-op physical. He was patient with me while I cried.

He was the only one who could get it through my thick skull that I was not leaving the hospital that day. At the end of our conversation, he gave me a fatherly kiss on the forehead. With that bit of magic, I knew everything would be alright.

I spent the night in the hospital alone. After returning with my overnight bag, Louis stayed with me until the end of visiting hours, long enough to watch me drink yet another bowel prep. I had just done one of these preps for the colonoscopy the day before and had been on a liquid diet for four days straight. Was there anything left inside me? Apparently there was.

Intellectually, I knew what this surgery was going to entail: Dr. Quilici was going to cut out my sigmoid colon, remove the adjacent lymph nodes, and remove my left ovary in what would be a combination of laparoscopic and open surgery. The cyst and colon would be too large to remove through tiny incisions. The recovery would be difficult, so I should expect to stay in the hospital for several days.

The only good thing about living so far away from my best friend Lori is the time difference between New York and California. This allowed me to chat with her at 3:30 a.m. Her words reaching me during the darkest hours of the night kept me from losing my mind with fear. When the amazing night nurse, Lucia, who had checked on me maybe more often than was necessary, came by my room to tell me her shift was over, I hugged her with all the gratitude for the compassion she showed me coupled with the fierceness of love I owed Lori.

•   •   •   •   •

Thursday, December 9, 2021, I awoke from surgery to my new reality: I definitely have cancer.

For weeks, I had been living with that terrible feeling of knowing that something was wrong and not being able to put my finger on it. And the worst of those fears, the thing I did not want to believe was possible, had turned out to be true.

I awoke from anesthesia to horrifying pain and confusion. The recovery room nurse rushed to hit me with morphine. Amidst a flurry of activity to prepare me to be moved to my room, I reached out and grabbed the nurse's hand. Through the pain, I could focus only on her blurry face. I tried and failed to speak, my throat hurt and my brain was jumbled. She squeezed my hand and smiled kindly down at me as they rolled me away. I felt her fingers slip away from mine, the way the morphine let consciousness slip from me. I returned to the wondrous place where there was no more pain or much of anything at all.

The next 12 hours come back to me as disjointed flashes of consciousness: Louis standing over me, kissing my face and petting my hair, and my voice in the distance saying to him, "I had so many dreams..." An unfamiliar man's voice: "Can you slide yourself into the bed?" The sensation of being lifted and moved from the gurney onto the hospital bed followed by a grunt which probably came from me. A woman's gentle voice asked, "Are you squeamish?" Louis' nervous response, "No." A soft hand lifted my hospital gown.

Louis did a lot of crying, a lot of kissing me, cradling my hand in his, and petting my hair. Clearly, I got the better end of this deal; the morphine kept me just slightly out of touch with consciousness. Louis, on the other hand, was wide awake and feeling everything for the both of us.

While I was drifting in and out of the merciful morphine dreams, Louis was bombarded with scary information. To his credit, he never told me what my staging was, and kept to himself the full details of what he had learned in the conversation he had with Dr. Quilici while I was in recovery. Not until January, after I had started chemotherapy and was reading over the notes from my hospital stay, did I discover I had Stage-4 Colon Cancer. And it was not until I finished radiation half a year later that Louis reluctantly told me the complete story.

Dr. Quilici informed him that the cancer, which I had interpreted at the time to mean *one tumor*, was instead a sticky mess inside my pelvis. This made it impossible for him to remove more because there was no space to negotiate the surgical tools inside me. He had removed over six inches of my large intestine and part of my peritoneal sac, along with the left ovary. But if he had tried to remove all the cancer he saw, I would have lost my rectum and likely my vagina as well. He opted for a colostomy, and to let chemotherapy have a shot at the remaining disease.

Whether my new colostomy would be permanent depended on if Dr. Quilici needed to remove my rectum after chemotherapy. No rectum, no reversal. The assumption was that the disease would cause extensive damage, and he was nearly certain that I would keep the colostomy for life. But until I found the courage to look objectively at the situation, I would not understand that the doctors did not expect me to live long enough to discuss a reversal. Dr. Quilici was doing me a kindness by giving me this small thing to hope for.

Louis asked Dr. Quilici how long I might survive after this. Did he think I had a couple of months? A couple of years? Dr. Quilici mercifully responded, "Don't think in numbers." It seemed he wanted to impress upon Louis that a cancer diagnosis was not an automatic death sentence. How in the world did Louis find the courage to ask that question? I never thought to ask it of anyone, because obviously I was not going to die.

For once, blissful ignorance was useful, sparing me the dark reality of how bad the situation actually was.

I was lucid enough to almost hold a conversation in the late evening. Louis wanted to know how I was feeling, and if was I having any pain. I responded: "Fuuuuuuck this shiiiiiiit."

He started laughing, his release of the intense fears and anxieties of the last few hours and months. He texted Lori: "Her first words after she woke up were 'fuck this shit'." Lori texted back, "She's going to be just fine."

Excruciating pain tortured me through the night — I was getting morphine every three hours to keep me unconscious. But the moment the drug wore off, I awoke to blinding pain. I could not speak. I could not think. Nothing existed in my world except **The Pain**. Between gaps in a strange sound (Louis told me I was making a horrible noise), I heard the night nurse tell me I would have to wait another hour before receiving more morphine. Unacceptable. Louis called the floor nurse. If he had not been there, that nurse would have made me wait out that hour in agony. And without his persistence, we would not have discovered that the pain management instructions listed in my chart was "on demand." He should not have had to beg for my relief. In the early morning hours, though, the worst of the pain had passed. They could lower me down to other medications for pain control. "Bye morphine. I'll miss you…"

I spent five days in the hospital recovering from the surgery. They gave Louis permission to stay with me every night. I was delighted to have him close by, and thankful he had been there to advocate for pain management. Later, we would come to find out the policy only allowed parents of small children or spouses of terminal patients to stay. He was not there because they bent the rules for us. He was there because my situation was grim.

Friday afternoon, 24 hours post-op, the expectation was that I would get out of bed and walk one lap of the ward. It was on this walk that Nurse Lou told me a bit about her ileostomy. She told me that even though things looked scary now, I would get used to the colostomy. Before I knew it, I would be back to have it reversed. Her ileostomy was not supposed to be reversible, but she kept a positive attitude and a year later, she had that reversal. She was living a completely normal life now. If such a tough case can be reversed, then so can my completely routine descending colostomy. She told me to remember that I was in the best surgical hands around. If Dr. Quilici says it is reversible, then it is.

But on that day, I was in no mood to talk about reversals. I wanted to pretend my colostomy did not exist. No force in the universe could make me look at it. As far as I was concerned, this was not my problem. I sure as hell was not ok with it. If I never saw it with my own eyes, then it did not exist.

I imagine women with breast cancer who have had mastectomies feel the same about that procedure as I did about my colostomy: a mixture of anger, curiosity, fear, relief, frustration, and hope. I had something cut from my body to save my life, and yet there I was resisting giving the owed gratitude to the thing. It was a mixed emotional reminder of the battle I fought for my life.

Lou gave me an even greater gift by focusing my attention on *when* and not *if*. She was so certain that after chemotherapy, I *would* be back in the hospital for a reversal, that I had no other option than to believe her. Not a single doubt in my mind that her subtle language was critical to my survival. I adopted her perspective immediately. *When I'm done with chemotherapy* (which, of course, will work perfectly because why would it not?), *I will have the reversal.*

Friday morning, the day after surgery, I was already wide awake when Dr. Jacobs, my new oncologist, appeared at the foot of my bed at the late hour of 5:30 a.m. I knew what he was going to tell me. By the time the words *Colon Cancer* came out of his mouth, I had already made peace with the whole thing. *Yes, I know. I guess I've always known.* He was reassuring, kind, and crackling with positive energy, which I found incredible. I have known many oncologists. They are not exactly famous for their warmth of personality. Surrounded day in and day out by people who are facing death with varying odds, I have found them to be morose, a little too forthcoming, and always a bit emotionally distant. Dr. Jacobs was refreshingly the opposite. He was exactly the kind of person I needed.

My leg cuffs inflated and deflated quietly in the background. I tried to measure my breathing against their rhythm to stay present in the conversation. "These kinds of tumors tend to dissolve with this particular chemotherapy regimen we're going to use." *Dissolve! I like that word!*

"And if anything is left of the tumor after chemotherapy, Dr. Quilici will remove it when he reverses your colostomy." But what I heard was, "One way or another, we'll get this stuff out of you and put you back together again."

Dr. Quilici advised Louis not to think in numbers. He did not want him to focus on cancer stages and statistics. This was important for both of us to remember, because my diagnosis was fucking scary: Aggressive Malignant Neoplasm of the Sigmoid Colon, Stage-4C.

The results of the pathology:
Colonoscopy biopsy: negative
12cm of the Sigmoid Colon removed, along with 20 adjoining lymph nodes, 6 of which tested positive for cancer

2 random sample lymph nodes of the abdomen tested negative
13cm[9] ovary, removed: benign
3cm ovarian mass: colon cancer
Cancerous tumor present on the outer rectum wall remains intact

The unique thing about my situation is that the cancer was *outside* the colon, not inside it. This explained the negative colonoscopy biopsy. It had spread over several inches of the outside of the sigmoid colon, jumped to six of the adjoining lymph nodes, the peritoneal wall, and the ovary, creeping through me like some 1950s' sci-fi gooey blob monster. Even if the doctor had been able to do the colonoscopy, he would not have seen this cancer. It was because an entire team of doctors came together that they solved this mystery in time to save my life.

Dr. Jacobs reminded us that surgeons are not magicians. Sometimes it is not possible to remove all the malignancies that they see without causing more damage. In my case, this was true. Dr. Quilici had thought long and hard during surgery about what would be the best way to proceed. He reassured Louis that he did not come to this decision lightly. Quality of life was an important factor. He felt that leaving the cancer on my rectum in place, then attempting to shrink — hopefully eradicate — it with chemotherapy, was my best option.

We asked about the use of the term *aggressive* with this cancer, and he explained that fast-dividing cells can be more susceptible to interruption by chemo than slow-dividing cells. Although *aggressive cancer* sounds scary, it can make it easier for chemo to do its job, so ironically it is good news.

[9] Roughly the size of a grapefruit

"Don't worry. This is all temporary." Dr. Jacobs reached down and squeezed my foot through the blanket in a most reassuring and kind way, casting his spell over me. From this moment forward, I would take whatever medicine Dr. Jacobs prescribed and I would do whatever he said to do. I would follow him to the ends of the earth.

·　　·　　·　　·　　·

On Monday, December 13, four days after my surgery, I went home. I needed a few days to rest, to recover, and to wrap my brain around the whole situation before meeting with Dr. Jacobs for the first official consultation. His assistant, Alex, called me Tuesday morning to set up the appointment; they had an opening for the next day, but I told her I was not emotionally ready to see him yet. She said she completely understood. Would Friday morning be better?

For a few extra days, I could ignore the cancer thing. I would not have to think about it or worry about it. If I wanted, I could pretend I was perfectly healthy again.

Willful ignorance can only last so long. We met with Dr. Jacobs on Friday morning, one-week post-op, to discuss my treatment plan. I was told I would get a chemotherapy called FOLFIRINOX,[10] a combination of drugs that was highly effective in treating this type of colon cancer. I would have these aggressive and powerful drugs in six doses over 12 weeks. They would monitor me every week (blood tests, basic check-ups) during treatment. We would begin as soon as Dr. Quilici could install the portacath in my chest, aiming for the first week of January. This meant I had almost four solid weeks to prepare. I

---

[10] The drugs in this therapy are: Leucovorin, 5-Fluorouracil (5-FU), Irinotecan and Oxaliplatin. For more information: https://www.cancer.gov/about-cancer/treatment/drugs/folfirinox

had lost 16 pounds up to this point, so my primary job was to put back as much of that weight as I could and to exercise. I needed to keep my body in top condition before being knocked down with the chemotherapy.

I believe there are subtle messages that come to us if only we open ourselves up to listen. After awakening from surgery, I found I was a much more open conduit than I had ever been in my life. An important message reached me in a waking dream state in the form of a very real voice whispering in my ear. "A demon needs to give up its name in order to be exorcised. This tumor needs to give up its name in order to be destroyed." I took this to heart.

So, I asked Dr. Jacobs, "What's the name of the tumor?"

He simply responded: "It's just your basic, run-of-the-mill, colon cancer. Nothing fancy."

I liked the sound of that. A powerless name.

This not-fancy, basic, run-of-the-mill colon cancer did not stand a chance.

THE CONE

In 2016, just a couple of months after my beloved cat, Dusty, passed away from stomach cancer, we adopted three dogs from a rescue in the high desert outside of Los Angeles. We never planned on adopting three dogs. We only planned to adopt one dog, but it turns out Louis is an even bigger softie than I am when it comes to hard-luck doggies.

While searching for adoptable dogs on the *Beagles and Buddies* website, I became distracted when the picture of a scruffy mutt named *Dusty* popped up on my screen. "This has to be a sign, right?" I knew Louis would see it my way: the Universe was sending me a replacement *Dusty*. I seem to remember Louis muttering, "Uh-oh."

The next morning, I called the rescue and arranged for us to meet Dusty the Dog that weekend. "He has a sister who also needs a home." The helpful voice was bubbling with optimism. "We think they should be adopted out together." She sent me Luna's profile. We had not met either dog yet, but it was obvious from their pictures they were both coming home with us.

Two dogs? Sure, why not. I had never had a dog before. How hard could two dogs be?

When we met Luna a few days later, Dusty was nowhere to be seen. Luna was very shy. The staff told me she never let people pet her, which was why this beautiful dog had not yet been adopted. It was instantly clear that she would not be like that with me! She rolled on her back and let me rub her belly. Then she did something there in the dirt that would become her signature show of affection with me over the years: pressing her forehead against mine and staring passionately into my eyes like a furry little paramour.

"Oh, we're taking her home," I said to the rescue director. It had not dawned on me yet that we had not met Dusty. Once he saw his sister following me around the enclosure, though, he became curious and materialized out of the crowd of 30 other dogs.

Dusty and his sister are Basenji-Cockapoo mixes. Sounds exotic; they look like miniature wolfhounds with the same basic body shape and wild, scruffy fur. Luna is deep graphite grey highlighted with silver and a white diamond on her chest. Dusty is a brindle, which is only obvious when we are lucky enough to get a glimpse of his speckled belly. Mostly his tangled fur makes him look like a feral street dog. Neither dog had been properly socialized as puppies, which explained their outright fear of people and resistance to being touched. Luna, the more manageable of the pair, had a bath in anticipation of our arrival that day. She was fancy — like a debutante. But Dusty was as wild as his filthy blond fur, and probably had never seen shampoo or a brush during his 22 months on the planet.

Engrossed with Dusty and Luna, I had not noticed what was going on by Louis. A small, senior beagle-dachshund mix with cloudy eyes and no teeth named Miles, had planted himself at Louis' heel and would not let him out of his sight. My turn to say "Uh-oh." We were smitten with this strange little pack of misfits, and a few hours later, we were carting this ragtag group of defective dogs back to our house.

Have I mentioned I had never had a single dog before this?

Over the next few years, we had multiple dog trainers working with Dusty and Luna to teach them how to walk on a leash. They had to learn how to do the most basic normal dog things. Luna succeeded, blossoming into a sweet and sensitive dog. Dusty, on the other hand, became so bonded to me it borders on a psychosis. I did not take this role lightly, so I used it to help him become more adventurous and curious about the world. Ironically, despite how frightened and stressed he is all the time (we mostly control his anxiety with Prozac), he is actually quite brave and loves to explore the hiking trails. He even enjoys going to the vet. This dog will do anything, as long as he does it with me. He also bonded closely with the little beagle mix. Although Miles only lived for three years after we adopted him, he taught Dusty the ropes of how to be a normal dog.

Dusty and Luna are my constant companions. They showed me how to just *be* in a moment; to enjoy the feel of scrub brush rubbing against my legs on the trail; and how to lie in the grass, soaking up the mid-afternoon sun when I am supposed to be doing important human things.

Dusty taught me how to deal with the situation at hand without looking too far into the future and showed me how to celebrate life's little victories. "I am walking with the dogs," I would repeat to keep myself grounded when we took our first tentative steps together out the front door during our training sessions. He taught me not to wish for them to be any kind of dog other than the ones they are. They will never be normal dogs, and I am okay with that. These dogs had been training me all along.

In August 2021, around the time my intestinal symptoms were stealing the spotlight from the gynecological ones, Dusty injured himself in our backyard. He ran full speed past an old water spigot and sliced his leg. The wound split open in the most dramatic way; since there is no fat on this dog's body, I got a splendid view of his muscles through the giant hole. I felt guilty and panicky when we arrived at the veterinarian's office, I believed I had let him down by allowing him to get hurt. I had failed him. While I waited at home for the vet to call to tell me to pick him up after his surgery, I wrapped the spigot in an old towel, dog-proofed a few other questionable backyard dangers, and hoped that would be enough to keep both dogs safe from more injuries.

When I picked him up later that day, he was sporting the infamous cone of shame, with a dozen stitches stretching for two inches across his front leg. He looked like a stuffed animal repaired by a well-meaning mom. Over the next nine weeks, we would have those stitches twice replaced by staples. It took forever for the wound to heal. With the tight line of staples, he looked like he had a zipper on his leg.

I was way more upset by Dusty's physical state than he was. He could do all his normal daily dog things with the cone on. He seemed oblivious to the line of staples. He sat bravely while I slathered Manuka honey on his wound and then ran back to the yard to play rough with his sister. I was eager to get his staples removed so he could be free of the cone, and yet he did not seem to mind it at all. I only took it off for him to eat his meals. After he ate, I would hold it out to him. "Stick your neck in the cone." He would slowly walk toward me and, yes, lay his neck in the cone while I buckled it around him. The same dog that had lived in fear under an old bookcase at the dog rescue now seemed to enjoy performing the trick of putting on his cone.

Instead of constantly worrying about my pain and imagining the worst about my intestines, the steady schedule of vet appointments and constant care for Dusty kept me distracted. In those precious weeks before my diagnosis, I was learning a very important lesson from my dog about acceptance and coping with the immediate situation. Dusty was not sulking or feeling sorry for himself because he had to wear a cone. He showed no frustration each time the staples had to be replaced; three times the healing had to start over from square one. He was figuring out how to use the cone to block his sister from stealing his toys. He was not wasting precious energy counting down the days until the cone came off; he just knew that *today* he was sticking his neck in the cone.

Through all the months I dealt with cancer, I aspired to be like him whenever I got ahead of myself. If I thought about my next chemo treatment, or worse, fret about things that *might* happen weeks down the line, I would think about Dusty in the cone. "I'm doing *this* now. I don't have to think about what might happen next month." It allowed me to be present with the side effects of chemo and radiation. His attitude would be the model for how I would view the colostomy. Instead of wishing I was healthy and there was no bag, I would think, "This is what's going on with my body now," and then sit with it. None of this is *fun*, but none of this is forever, either. I just have to stick my neck in the cone today, and maybe tomorrow its removal will surprise me.

Unexpectedly for both of us, Dusty received his reprieve from the cone one morning. I took it off so he could eat breakfast and never put it back on. He looked a little confused, staring up at me with his dark brown eyes, his curled tail wagging expectantly. He stood over the cone, which I had carelessly dropped on the kitchen floor, patiently waiting for me to pick it up and ask him to stick his neck in the cone again. It never happened; he was free.

I quickly forgot about the cone, lying there by the food bowls, as I started going about my usual morning routine. In the background, I kept hearing a strange noise, but I thought little of it. When I returned to the kitchen, I found a fantastic sight! Dusty had been busy shredding the plastic cone to pieces. And he was now sitting in the middle of the mess looking up at me, pleased as punch. I laughed, kissed his forehead, ruffled his fur, and praised him with an amused "Good boy!" while I cleaned up the mess.

He might have been stoic and brave all those weeks he wore the cone, but when it came down to it, his greatest pleasure was ripping it to pieces.

Because fuck that cone.

TULIP

I am not a doctor, but I watch a lot of them on tv. I am highly unqualified to give medical advice, despite my vast knowledge of make-believe medicine. Colon cancer has inspired me to learn more about actual medicine, anatomy, cancer treatments, statistics, and mental health effects. It has also gifted me a new perspective on just how little most of us know about cancer treatments, procedures, and medical jargon. We live without knowing just how common cancer all around us is.

Often, when I tell someone that I have cancer, they see a woman in her 40s and jump to the conclusion that I have breast cancer. When they find out I have colon cancer, they seem shocked. The insinuation is that somehow a woman cannot have colon cancer. Just because they make a big deal about their morning constitution, does that mean men are the only ones who have colons? I cannot believe that is true; the end of mine was sticking out of my abdomen. I found the reactions toward colon cancer to be fascinating, if not a bit sexist.

Colon cancer is not shameful. It does not represent some sort of failure on the patient's part. It is not something to be squeamish about. It is the third most common type of cancer[11]: men have about 1 in 23 (4.3%) risk, women have only a slightly lower risk at 1 in 25 (4.0%) risk. Just like every cancer, it is life-threatening. We need to fight it with every ounce of strength we have. It needs to be talked about even though it may not be flashy or sexy. This is a cancer that affects the most basic of our bodily functions. Having a hang-up over poop will save no one's life. Nor was it going to help me cope with the aftermath of a major surgery like a colectomy.

By the time my brush with colon cancer was over, I learned an important lesson: my body is not *me*. It is just a thing. And that thing needs to be healed. It cannot get its treatments if I am embarrassed about showing someone my butt. As this eventful year progressed, I shed all modesty about my back end, and I learned to laugh off just about every procedure that was done with it. I had fingers, enemas, scopes, and cameras stuck in my rectum, pen marks and stickers on my anus, and once a doctor examined it with an iPhone flashlight. ("I better not see that on the internet later!") Dropping my pants before each radiation treatment in front of three nurses was no big deal, and I even learned the best positions to help the doctors with their digital exams. After a while, it became just another body part the doctors needed unfettered access to. They were only doing their jobs, and they were not the ones feeling weird about any of it.

It was shocking to wake up to discover I had a colostomy. Like most people, I had never heard of this before other than vague references to "a bag" when talking about old people. I thought I did not know anyone who had one. When in fact, I knew two people who did. They just never talked about it. It's a very private matter. Rarely do people talk as openly as I did

[11] According to the National Cancer Institute, 2022 https://www.cancer.gov/types/common-cancers

while I had mine. According to the United Ostomy Associations of America (UOAA), over one million people in the United States are living with a colostomy[12]. So, chances are, unless they have an ostomy[13], most people are like I was — unaware of the hidden world of ostomates. Sometimes I felt like I was a part of the Wizarding World, but instead of secret magic wands, it was secret bags of poop.

I spared zero thoughts to the possibility of a colostomy, despite the nurses talking to me extensively about it the night before my surgery. It seemed obvious this would not happen to me. I believed Dr. Quilici was just going to sew me back up.

My colon cancer involved the sigmoid colon, the last twist before the rectum, which acts as a reservoir. That stretch of colon had to be removed during my surgery. It left me with what is called a Descending Colostomy, the descending colon being the last intact part of my large intestine before the stoma. My rectum, at the other end of the disconnected pipe, was still inside me, alive and healthy, but not attached to anything. The answer to everyone's burning question is yes, my rectum still worked, even though nothing except occasional mucus came out. Losing part of the colon is like losing a stretch of piping under the kitchen sink: sure, it is helpful to have the U-bend to catch all the food bits and gunk, but if it is not there, will the house burn down? After the surgeon removed the twisty bit of my intestine and sewed up the ends, I did not burst into flames either.

The morning after my colectomy, the surgical team congregated around the foot of my bed like little green men preparing to collect me for experiments on the mother ship. If

[12] https://www.ostomy.org
[13] Ostomy is a general term that refers to either colostomy (large intestine), ileostomy (small intestine), or urostomy (bladder) diversion

all four team members were there, then I could not expect good news. Still, nothing they said about the cancer would have surprised me at that point. Dr. Jacobs had already been in to see me.

I only had one concern: "When can I get back to my yoga practice?" Dr. Quilici let out a little laugh. "You have a 6-inch incision in your abdomen, young lady. Can you please wait for two weeks until I see you at your post-op check?" With a sly smile, I acquiesced. Perfect. That was all I needed to hear.

The colostomy was there; I knew it. Reaching under my hospital gown, I felt the appliance stuck to me. I just lacked the stomach to look at it. Plus, I was a little pissed off. The end of my colon is sticking out through my skin? They expect me to poop in a bag? The world has gone mad.

The colostomy was, by far, the biggest emotional hurdle in this theater of chaos. In so many ways, I was more upset about the colostomy than the cancer. The colostomy distracted me from the real problem (cancer) in the same way the cone distracted Dusty from the real problem (wound).

I cried a lot, bursting with anger and grief. Being squeamish, I do not handle blood well. I had already come up hard against my limit while taking care of Dusty's flesh wound. How could I be expected to look at an internal organ sticking out of my abdomen? It took me a while before I found the courage to look at the stoma. I was afraid that I might see something so gross, I would never be able to take care of myself on my own.

Nurse Lou to the rescue. She decided it was time for me to face reality and gave me the gentle encouragement I needed to lift my hospital gown and have a look. Turns out, my new stoma was not so bad. It looked like a little pink glob. "They call it a rosebud." She stood over me like a midwife standing over a new mother.

It looked more like a tulip. Naming my stoma *Tulip* had a positive effect on my mental well-being. And having such a sunny, feminine, hopeful name allowed me to see it for what it represented: *life.*

•   •   •   •   •

Living with a colostomy was not the end of the world. In my case, it barely rose to the level of an inconvenience. But it took several weeks for me to reach that point.

I figured I had four weeks between surgery and the start of chemotherapy during which I needed to get a handle on three things: recover from surgery, gain weight, and figure out this colostomy situation. I knew I could do it, but could I do it on my self-imposed timeline?

"You don't have to be perfect at it right away," Dr. Jacobs said to me the morning I was to be discharged from the hospital. "There's a learning curve."

With me, there is no such a thing as a learning *curve.* I work in straight lines from start to finish. Also, *right away* is my middle name. Dr. Jacobs did not know he had issued me a challenge. I was going to be the *best* colostomy patient he ever had. *You'll see. You'll all see!*

I was very lucky to have had Nurse Lou by my side in those early hours. She spoke frankly about the colostomy. Thanks to her experience with her ileostomy, she made me feel, right from the beginning that this was not something to be ashamed of or stressed about. "Think of it like changing a diaper," she counseled me. "The first few days after you brought home your newborn baby, it peed and pooped on you; you put the diaper on backward; there were leaks, and it fell off. But what happened after a couple of weeks? You became a diaper ninja." She was right: I was *the* Diaper Ninja back in my day.

Her positive attitude injected essential optimism and confidence into my situation. Very few people are this lucky to have their first introduction to the world of ostomies be this positive. Having a nurse with an ileostomy as my companion in the days immediately following surgery was kismet. I know that I would have had a positive attitude about it eventually. But without her, it would have taken much longer and the winding road would have been more like a crazy straw.

Once discharged from the hospital, I could begin my mental recovery. I joined an ostomy support group, where I learned potty jokes are a great way to cope with the situation. A never-ending stream of fart jokes kept the mood light at home, too. "What did that asshole say?" I would quip when a random fart would punctuate a serious sentence. "You say the most romantic things," Louis would coo while we cuddled in bed at night, a stream of gas bellowing from my new blowhole. We had fun with it. We had no other choice. Why not laugh about it?

Right away, I decided it was important for me to share this very private, unique, physical experience with everyone I knew. I wrote about it in my blog and talked about it openly with close friends and family. I showed it to anyone who wanted to see it. My friend Pam was dying for a peek. "I'll probably never see another one again," she said, enthusiastic, diving right in. I was happy that people wanted to be a part of this. If I had hidden it, if I had kept it a secret and gone through my entire cancer treatment telling no one about it, I would not have been quite as well adjusted as I was.

I had many moments, however, where I allowed myself to feel sorrow for the situation. It is complicated to explain to someone who has never had a significant medical change in their bodies. Unlike a bad haircut that would sort itself out in a few weeks or going out in a new pair of glasses for the first time, the stoma had a permanence about it. Getting the colostomy reversal would be like having breast reconstruction. Even though a woman *looks* like herself again, she will always be someone who had a mastectomy. I will always be someone who had a colostomy. There is no reversing that.

The colostomy became a part of my *cancer identity*. It was an outward symbol of the journey I was on. Chemo with a colostomy. Radiation with a colostomy. Cancer with a colostomy. Sometimes the colostomy was a sad visual reminder of the horrible situation of the cancer diagnosis, and other times when it said, "You are alive because of me."

Once I healed up from the colectomy surgery, around the two-week mark, and just as Dr. Quilici had predicted, I got back on the yoga mat with no limitations. Being fit and with strong abdominal muscles before the colostomy, I was at low risk for a parastomal hernia, something that is very common among ostomates. I had no problems with yoga, doing twists and inversions, abdominal strengthening exercises, and backbends. In fact, I could even lay on my stomach for things like Bow Pose while, incidentally, it was the portacath that prevented me from lying flat with my chest down. The only things I could not do were arm balances that required my elbows to dig into my abdomen. No matter. If I qualified for a reversal at the end of this, then I would have the rest of my life to do those poses again.

This is what I am doing now. I am sticking my neck in the cone today.

I took a lot of photos of myself doing complicated yoga poses with my colostomy bag hanging out for all the world to see. There was nothing to be ashamed of, and everything to be proud of. *I am thriving.* Despite all the physical setbacks leading up to this, I was still strong. And it always amused me that, despite having cancer, I was otherwise healthy. It would have been crazy to give up my fitness activities and feel sorry for myself the whole time. I believe that staying active helped me accept the colostomy faster and more completely.

I understood that within my support group, I was in the minority of people who came to accept their stoma and make peace with it. Since I cannot force people to see things my sunny way, I decided I would take it upon myself to model healthy living with an ostomy in a happy and positive way. I shared yoga and hiking photos. I engaged in as many conversations as I could, and whenever I sensed someone going down a dark path, I tried as best I could to support them. Everyone copes in different ways, but it pains me to see people who cannot find the positive in a situation.

What I observed, most times, was that the ostomate had been on the path to acceptance but came across roadblocks put up by people around them who did not understand the experience. They would project their own baseless insecurities onto the ostomate. Without a solid support system, no wonder so many ostomates struggle to come to accept their situation, it is nearly impossible to live with optimism under the shadow of shame. Louis gave me immense amounts of support by wanting to care for me and to learn all he could about the colostomy. He never looked at me differently, and even though he got poop on his hands a couple of times, this situation brought us even closer.

Yes, having a colostomy sucks big time. But there were so many good things that came out of it. I learned to have deeper empathy for people. I met new friends with ostomies. And I came to appreciate that there are many unique medical conditions out there that people avoid talking about. It all came down to just one simple yet astounding fact: *I'm alive*. Just that alone would help me shift my attitude whenever I felt myself slipping toward the dark side again.

Once I started chemotherapy, of course, I became focused on that, not so much on the colostomy anymore. Having achieved my self-imposed four-week goal, the colostomy faded into the background. I had a good handle on my diet. I wanted to know everything I could about the digestive process and the organs involved, learning fancy anatomical words like "cecum" and "distal." And I stopped worrying if people could see the bag under my clothes. We went out to dinner, and I wore tight jeans and my favorite shirts. Nurse Lou was right: I became a colostomy ninja. Like a one-woman pit-crew, I could change the whole appliance in less than five minutes before having to run out the door to an appointment. I could go to my infusions and not worry about what I would do if I had to empty my bag in the shared bathroom at the cancer center. During radiation, I had no hang-ups about laying on the treatment table with the bag showing for all the technicians to see. My motto was "It's not rocket science, it's a bag of crap."

After all those months with the colostomy, I became very fond of my stoma and even felt gratitude toward it. In May 2022, I had had it for only five months, but I already had mixed feelings about the possibility of losing the colostomy going into the next surgery after chemotherapy. The next scheduled procedure sought to remove whatever remained of the tumor on my rectum and to assess if a takedown of the colostomy was possible. I list them in this order because the most important part of the surgery was the exploratory portion — to see what the chemotherapy had accomplished. All I knew for sure was that I would awaken to find out if I would need more treatment.

I felt the appliance still stuck to my abdomen when I awoke from that surgery, giving me all the instant feedback I required. The reversal had not happened, which I understood meant Dr. Quilici saw more cancer inside of me. But I also understood something else: I was not feeling sadness about my situation. In just those short five months, I had done all the difficult mental work to make peace with and accept my colostomy. If it was going to be permanent, I would be ok. I had added *Colostomy Ninja* to my resume. And most important of all, I knew everyone still loved me, with or without the colostomy.

I expected I would stop talking about the colostomy as it assimilated into my daily life. Everything would be ok. I was ok. I was alive. And who cares about the colostomy? Not me. As a result, I resolved to reach out more, help more people, and become even more active in the ostomy community. I might not be able to do it while going through treatment; but I thought, *when I'm better,* I will make this my mission.

After the surgery, Dr. Quilici told me the colostomy could be reversed, the tissues were healthy enough, and we would try again in a few months after I completed radiation. I was looking at another five months with the colostomy. That did not seem so daunting. In fact, it was a non-issue for me. I was more afraid of the upcoming radiation treatments and all the unknowns that go along with that. The colostomy remained the outward sign that I was still going through treatments. My hair might grow back, but the colostomy would remain unchanged. As long as the colostomy was there to remind me I was still in this fight, I would show gratitude for every extra day that it afforded me.

For all these months, I had done the hard work to accept the colostomy. I was prepared to wear the cone forever if I needed to. I just had to remember that it was because of *Tulip* that I was still alive.

I got this whole thing in the bag.

PART TWO

"I feel thin, sort of stretched,
like butter scraped over too much bread."
— *Bilbo Baggins*

FOLFIRITRON

Upon arriving home from the hospital five days after the colectomy, the lure of a hot shower helped keep my mind off the scary diagnosis. There would be no erasing reality with a scrub down, but I would still try. My hair was greasy from five days of not washing, my skin coated in a layer of dried sweat, my teeth felt furry, and I was pretty certain I smelled like I had been living in a van down by the river. Cancer could wait. I needed to start over with a good lather and lots of steam.

I had lost 12 pounds leading up to surgery. Cancer is a ravenously hungry disease, lacking self-control. It will greedily devour its host. I also knew that after four days on a controlled liquid diet in the hospital, I could expect more weight loss. I had not seen my body in a mirror for close to a week since there had been no reason to be naked in my hospital room. To top it off, I wore an oversized hospital gown the entire time. The only parts of my body I had seen were my arms, and they were not looking particularly meaty. I worried about what was under the rest of my clothes now.

Louis had to help me with my first shower. The 6-inch incision connecting my belly button to my pubic bone was still raw. We made a lame attempt at covering it to keep the sutures dry. The new colostomy bag felt garish, hanging off me like a deflated extra lung. I was operating with deep fatigue. I worried about my ability to stand long enough to take a shower at all. While Louis was covering my incisions with waterproof dressings, I could not take my eyes off my reflection in the mirror. I looked like a poorly drawn stick figure version of myself. The tops of my thighs did not touch anymore. I could count all my ribs, and my face looked drawn and pale. My head balanced precariously on top of an unnaturally thin body I did not recognize. Louis undressed and turned on the water to heat it up.

"I'm going to hop on the scale really quick." The numbers lit up on the scale's digital screen. Four more pounds gone, bringing the total to 16. I could not stop staring at the number. It seemed unreal. I think I was in junior high the last time I weighed this. "It's ok," Louis said, helping me into the tub. "We'll get you fattened up before you know it!" I wished I shared his optimism because at that moment everything seemed impossible: lifting my leg over the lip of the tub, washing my hair, pooping in a bag, beating this cancer, gaining weight.

Twelve weeks of chemotherapy loomed on the horizon. And then what? We knew nothing about the chemotherapy drugs I was about to have; I still thought Dr. Quilici had left behind just *one tumor* for the chemo to treat. My body was so frail I could not imagine it capable of enduring the massive drugs that would soon be pumped into it. How in the world was I going to get through this? It took every ounce of strength to prevent myself from dissolving into the steam; I struggled to hold my atoms together.

I had to lather up my hair twice. It was so filthy. Yet, an amazing thing was happening: a space was opening in my chest, allowing me to breathe again. Louis watched me like a hawk, ready to catch me if I looked as if I would slip, while he secretly rearranged my shampoos on the bench in case I needed to sit. Slowly, I felt myself coming back together. I was being reassembled and patched up with pear-scented, organic, not-tested-on-animals soap bubbles. I was exhausted, and yet here I was functioning on plenty of reserves. Maybe I was stronger than I thought.

I did not feel fear or sadness. I was not overwhelmed or powerless. I felt... nothing. I did not cry. I did not moan. I did not complain. My knees looked knobby, and I could see my hip bones sticking out, but this little body was to be my partner in this next battle. In yoga, we talk about the mind-body-spirit connection, and while we are healthy, I think most of us, myself included, make a fair attempt to understand what that means. In times of mortal danger, like cancer, the true meaning comes into sharp focus.

I was a team of three distinct *me's* preparing for this fight — body, mind, and spirit. *We* would have to learn to play nice together if *we* were going to get out of here alive.

So what if my *body* was underweight? Look at those muscles in my arms and abdomen and legs. They can carry me. My body was ready.

My *mind* was all over the place. But if I could get this wildcard to focus on a singular goal, it would be a powerful tool to navigate the rough waters ahead.

My *spirit* seemed to have its act together, with no instruction. I could feel the will to live and survive surging through me. It was never in question, and it never faltered.

I am going to live.

I did not just say it to soothe myself or anyone else. I felt it in my bones. There would be no other outcome except survival.

This would not be a battle; this was going to be a slaughter. *Cancer, you just tangled with the wrong bitch.*

Regardless of my seemingly heroic stance on facing cancer, and all the support I was receiving from friends and family, I felt very much alone and separated from everyone around me. I was living in a parallel dimension where I was the only one who existed under cancer's shadow. No one else could understand how I was feeling. I was not resentful or wistful; I just accepted it. *I have cancer now.* It was ok if Louis or Andrew had to sit back and observe my process. They should be thankful they had no clue what was going on inside of me. Sometimes I felt entitled to marinate in a little self-pity. I believed I deserved that indulgence before the real fight began.

Doing simple things around the house was done *with cancer.*

I am washing dishes *with cancer.*

I am watching tv *with cancer.*

I am walking down the hall *with cancer.*

I felt out of touch. I was looking at the world through a backward spyglass.

I was a lot of things during this time. But I was not dying. Of that, I was certain. I had nothing concrete or scientific to base this feeling on. I just *knew* it.

Keeping lock step with my every move, an actual Army had assembled behind me. From the moment I opened my eyes in the hospital, Lori, Ella, and Pam were at my side. They were the only people, other than Louis and Andrew, who knew all the details of what was going on with me ahead of my diagnosis. Now, they were leading the emotional charge. Each one held me up in their own essential way, preparing me for the fight. I leaned on them heavily during this time, and it touched me how quickly and naturally they rallied, found their purpose, and jumped to action.

One more soldier was going to be added to this tight little circle: Alice. As soon as the word got out about my diagnosis, a mutual friend of ours decided I needed her. A 10-year colon cancer survivor living in New York City, Alice's persistence and warmth broke through the miles and my defenses. She became a lifeline, her texts magically appearing on my phone screen at moments when I felt particularly intense emotions. She was always there, cheering me on, and sharing her journey with me.

These four women, each holding on to one of my limbs, propelled my every step like I was their well-worn marionette.

Now that I was home, the real recovery from surgery could happen; it was time to eat and prepare for chemotherapy. The only advice Dr. Jacobs gave me was, "Put on as much weight as you can." He also wanted me to get back on the yoga mat and the hiking trails as soon as possible. I needed to prepare my body for the onslaught of drugs headed its way. Exercise would be crucial to my recovery and preparations for chemo, and Dr. Jacobs and Dr. Quilici were very specific in telling me to resume my normal routines.

I was naïve thinking that gaining that much weight would be fun. My experience had always been that I could gain 3 pounds by just looking at a holiday cookie tray, so I figured it would be easy to gain it now. Eat all the food I want and gain back all the weight. No problem! It was hardly that simple, though.

No rule exists that says that all vegans are skinny; we gain weight just as easily as with any other lifestyle. But I was coping with the aftermath of a major abdominal surgery. I had lost half of a foot of my colon and was learning to live with the colostomy. My guts were not ready for me to dive into a normal menu. They were just learning to work again. The nutritionist at the hospital had given me very specific dietary instructions to follow while the colostomy healed. For the first week, I had to follow a *soft solids* diet, which slowly introduced foods one at a time to see how my gut reacted. I was told to avoid things like beans and ancient grains, which are high in the protein and calories that I needed to gain weight, but also high fiber, so at that early stage of recovery, verboten.

Although it would make gaining weight difficult, I decided to cut added sugar from my diet. The anecdotal evidence out there convinced me that feeding sugar to the cancer was not a great idea. They would be giving me one of the chemotherapy drugs in a solution of glucose. Why? To *bait* the cancer into consuming the drug. Kind of like putting the heart worm medicine into a glob of peanut butter to trick my dogs into eating the pills. I theorized that cutting sugar would starve the cancer, making it so desperate for sustenance that when the glucose laced chemicals appeared, it would greedily devour its own poison. It did not matter to me if it worked. Going sugar-free made me feel as if I was doing something on my own to stunt the cancer's growth before treatments began.

Louis and I kept a food diary to add up all the calories I was eating throughout the day and to see which eating patterns were most conducive to weight gain. With only four weeks to get the job done, we were on a tight deadline. It was a race between my body and the cancer to see which one could gobble up the calories first. We discovered I had to eat five times per day, adding up to 3500 calories daily to gain one solid pound per week. It sounds like it would be a lot of fun: eat whatever I want, all the time. But it was very tiresome for me. I was feeling sick and exhausted from eating so much and frustrated at not seeing much weight gain. By the time I started chemo, I had gained back four pounds. That was four pounds better than nothing.

During my free time between meals, I had to resist researching anything to do with the cancer I had or the chemotherapy I would receive. I also avoided poking around too much in the hospital patient portal that held all my medical information, test results, and pathology, including my diagnosis and the cancer staging. Lori decided she would do all the research on my behalf and only inform me on a *need-to-know* basis, much as I had done a few years earlier when her mother had been going through cancer treatments. It did not go unnoticed that Lori had decided there was not much I needed to know, while also keeping from me how worried she was about the outcome.

"It was gut-wrenching," she admitted months later when chemo was shrinking in the rearview mirror, "knowing how quickly your saga could have gone sideways."

Louis never showed it around me, but I could feel the waves of concern and worry radiating off him. Too many nights, he was lying awake at 2 a.m., ready to soothe me when I could not sleep. It seems he also spent the wee hours imagining all the terrible things that were about to happen to me. His voice would reach me through the darkness, whispering the words that would become an important mantra in the coming months: *don't be afraid of the chemo, be afraid of the cancer.*

During these weeks before chemo, I had many intense and realistic dreams, the kind that made me wonder if they were even dreams at all. I would spend hours, every day, writing down those dreams, going back through them, and trying to decipher their deeper meaning. Some I would not come to understand until months later, while others were clear messages I needed to hear to prepare for the coming storm. I took none of these messages lightly. During chemo, I would draw guidance and strength from one dream in which a faceless scientist showed me how a cancer cell dissolved with a drop of chemo. I would use this vision as meditation, envisioning the cancer cells in my body doing the same. The chemo had to work, it just *had to*. And I was convinced the power of my mind was going to help the drugs along.

To say that I *made peace* with my situation is not altogether correct. I was not freaking out or panicking. I was not protesting or bargaining with the Universe to make this go away. Because I knew for a fact that *I have cancer*. It was as real as real can get. There was no changing that. No wishing it away, no pretending it did not exist. No use in avoiding thinking about it. This is what acceptance feels like.

I have cancer.

So, Lisa, what will you do about it? Cry and hide or stand and fight? I may have been quiet and introspective during this period, and of course I had moments where I questioned my ability to face this disease head-on, but I was feeling strong, and sometimes I even felt a little bit brave.

I was ready. Bring on *The Abdominable*.

All my doctors, and all the nurses, never wavered in their optimism about my chances of surviving this cancer. There was no alternative. *I am going to live.* Dr. Jacobs spoke with great authority on the effectiveness and success of the chemotherapy drugs, using definitive statements like "*When* this is over." Dr. Kagan also remained optimistic: "Before you know it, we'll be toasting to your good health." They gave me no reason to think that there was another outcome besides a full recovery. They would pump *the poison cure* into me soon enough, and when they spoke like this, I believed anything was possible. This is so crazy that it just might work.

Despite all the optimism Louis and the doctors were showering upon me, it took just one nurse to throw a wrench into my delicate positivity machine. Twenty-four hours before chemo was to begin, I had surgery to have the portacath implanted in my chest, the internal device through which they would administer the chemotherapy. The pre-op admission process was going smoothly. After they weighed me, I changed into another extra-large hospital gown; the phlebotomist inserted the IV into my arm, and I met with the friendly anesthesiologist.

Enter Nurse Negative Nancy. Inputting my health information into the computer, she saw my recent Colon Cancer diagnosis. She said, "You probably have another 10 or 15 years after this," in the same casual tone with which a nurse might say, "I'll be back to draw more blood in 10 or 15 minutes."

What? She had hit me over the head with a sledgehammer. I was stunned. I had no response. Pretty sure I just said, "Uh-huh," and tried to ignore whatever else it was she was pontificating about. The worst part was that she said it softly enough that Louis did not hear it, making me question whether I had imagined the whole thing. My hard-earned emotional balance was teetering, and if I was not careful, this could poison my mind for the entirety of my treatment. I resented her. Over the next few months, her words crept back into my head. Sometimes, I struggled to find the strength to push them back out.

Ten or 15 more years to live? I'm only 47. Dead at 60? I'll show her. I'm going to live to be 100, just to rub it in her face.

The port surgery was quick and simple. I went home a couple of hours later starving and full of energy. I did not expect to sleep much that night, between the volts of electricity running through my body and the thrill of expectation of what was coming in the morning.

•   •   •   •   •

Wednesday, January 5, 2022. I was already wide awake when Louis' alarm went off at 5:00 a.m., the trumpet fanfare heralding the march to battle against the awaiting dragon, *The Abdominable.*

Ella had given me the very important advice to eat breakfast before my infusion, "Because if you throw up, you want something to throw up. And if you don't, it could be the last good meal you eat for a few days." I did not get creative with my last meal. I just had a chocolate protein shake. Turns out, she was right: I did not throw up, but it was the last solid thing I ate for the next three days.

Dressing was a thoughtful process. The shirt I chose had buttons. This would give the nurses easy access to the gross new portacath. I pulled on a cozy pair of fleece-lined leggings, the *Fuck Cancer* rainbow unicorn socks Lori had sent me, my un-ironic leg warmers, and the blue sparkle sneakers Louis had given me for Christmas the year before. I looked like a kindergartener wearing all my favorite clothes at once on the first day of school.

Into my day bag went the pink plush smiley-face colon from my cousin, a 32-oz bottle of water, my copy of *Harry Potter and the Sorcerer's Stone* (I figured light reading was the best companion for the heavy 12-week chemotherapy regimen), my iPad, charging cables, and colostomy supplies. I even tossed in a few snacks for Louis. I knew he was so focused on me he would not think to bring anything for himself.

The morning had all the excitement of the start of a long road trip toward my impending execution. The dogs could feel the tension in the air — they were not interested in their breakfast. Luna hid in my yoga-slash-music room, and Dusty, suspicious that something was out of the ordinary, stared at me from the dark hallway, one paw held up.

Too numb to think about much of anything, I navigated the morning on autopilot. I went about my packing checklist in silence, fearing if I spoke, I might snap at Louis, who, in no way, deserved any of my ire. We brushed our teeth, grabbed our bags, Andrew hugged me for good luck, and we walked through the door into the early morning half-light.

When I stepped off the front porch and onto the path to the driveway, the Cooper's hawk, who had built her nest in a tree in front of our house, swooped low across my path, causing me to stop short. She passed close enough that I could hear the air swooshing through her wings. This hawk would remain with me for the next 10 months, throughout the entirety of my treatments: calling to me from the tree beside our driveway when I arrived home from treatments, flying aerobatics through our backyard while I napped on the patio, and sitting in branches above my head as I laid in the grass with the dogs. Once she flew straight at me, pulling up just an arm's length from my face, flaring her feathers and hanging, suspended, in a glorious display. She was a powerful ally. I was never alone with her around.

For a moment, we were both paralyzed. "Definitely a good sign," Louis decided, opening the car door for me. I climbed in, astounded by my first up close and personal brush with the hawk. I was silent for quite some time, listening instead to Louis' encouraging and soothing chatter as he drove us out of the neighborhood.

The 30-minute car ride from Chatsworth to Burbank passed all too quickly. Los Angeles morning traffic is always curiously clear when I do not want to be somewhere.

There is a unique atmosphere in the Cancer Center at 7:00 a.m. compared to during normal business hours. The only people there, besides the doctors and nurses, were other patients awaiting their treatments. Two other people joined us in the elevator. The man looked brightly around at everyone. "So, what are you in for?" He bounced on the balls of his feet like a little boy.

"Breast cancer," the woman said. Both their eyes fell on me.

Hey! Louis is bald. Why don't they assume he's the one here for chemo? "Colon cancer," I answered. My indignation dissipated when the man revealed he had Chronic Lymphocytic Leukemia (CLL). I had just been initiated into a Cancer Tribe.

The woman left the elevator on the third floor, the women's cancer center, while the man rode to the top floor, the fourth floor, with us. They would be my first taste of the kinship among the patients at the Disney Family Cancer Center. Over the coming year, I would come to crave these interactions with other patients. And, I would soon discover I had become the *Ambassador* in the elevator.

After my requisite blood work and checkup with Dr. Jacobs, they directed me to the waiting room for the infusion center, which shared the fourth floor with his department. Several other patients were already waiting. The newbie with the furrowed brow took a seat. I felt all their eyes pass over me. I was the only person who still had all their hair. My mind flashed back to the little boy with the broken arm. Now I was the one expecting a monster behind the scary door waiting to gobble me up. Not knowing what horrors awaited me through the heavy wooden door with no windows, I was bracing for the unknown.

My eyes darted from the row of elevators to the empty nurses' desk to the clock above the water cooler and back around the horn again.

I tried not to stare at the other patients, though I felt a deep sense of camaraderie, empathy, and curiosity. Some people looked tired but otherwise ok, while others looked crumpled and transparent. Part of me wondered which camp I would fall into and how quickly that would happen. Another part of me made a pinky swear I would not suffer. *I want to be that person who they all look at and can't believe is having chemo;* I promised myself.

There was an important common thread to the advice given to me by Ella, Alice, and Dr. Jacobs: "You won't know how it's going to go until you're in it." No one could tell me how I was going to react to these drugs. Even if they had shared their side effects with me ahead of my treatments, it would not have mattered. Everyone is unique. Every drug is unique. Even different combinations of the drugs create unique experiences.

Unceremoniously, the door opened, and Odalys called everyone in. The others walked straight through the door unaccompanied, but Odalys welcomed me for my first treatment and led me through the door. She passed me on to one of the waiting nurses, who gave me a quick tour of the ward. My anxiety of the unknown easing with each new friendly face. I chose the bright corner room at the far end.

The infusion center boasts two walls of solid windows opening out to a view of Disney Studios across the street and nearby Griffith Park in the Santa Monica Mountains. Although bright, the winter sun never showed its full face through the glass. This meant that those of us whose drugs prevented us from being in the sunlight could leave our shades open the entire day if we desired. My drugs would make me one of those people. Toward the end of my treatments, I would be tired of hiding in the dark. I would crave the sun and the warmth of sunlight on my skin. I would need to see the world outside of every window of every building I was in. I was so desperate not to feel locked away that I would open the blinds in exam rooms and stare out the window at the dirty air conditioning units on rooftops below while I waited for doctors to meet with me.

My infusion nurse that day, Terry, was as sunny as the light through the windows as she described how the day would progress. Still, my brain refused to grasp the concept that the infusion would take over six hours. She had to repeat this multiple times. She walked me through the process. But she might as well have been speaking gobbledygook; the information coming at me with overwhelming speed. She said, "After today, you'll be an expert on your chemotherapy."

With her skilled hand, she accessed my brand new portacath that was still sore from surgery the day before and hooked me up to the two bags which she had already hung from my IV tree. The first drugs dripped into me. I wondered what the immediate effects would be. Would I be nauseous? Would my face swell up from the steroids? What was this *cold sensitivity* Terry was talking about? Would I be ill tonight, tomorrow, or ever? What mysterious and terrible side effects awaited me in my immediate future?

For the first hour, I felt pretty good. Although low-grade anxiety still bubbled under the surface, I was cocky: this chemo thing was not so bad. I had built it up to be Godzilla, but it was just a fence lizard. *Piece of cake!* Of course, they had only given me an anti-nausea medication and some saline.

Calls of "Chemo check!" periodically rang through the infusion center as other patients received their drugs throughout the morning. An hour into my infusion, Terry called "Chemo check!" again. This time, she appeared from behind my curtain, bringing with her my first drug, Leucovorin. The little bag sat on a tray along with some very serious-looking paraphernalia. With a quick scan of my wristband and verbal confirmation of my name and birthdate with a second nurse as a witness, chemotherapy began. She hung the small bag from my IV tree, connected the secondary line to a port on the primary tubing, and opened the valve. My heart rate skyrocketed as genuine fear coursed through my body and mixed with the drug. Between the other two clear bags, the new, small bag looked ominous, covered in its brown ultraviolet shield.

Eventually, I could calm down enough to continue reading my book. Although Louis stayed with me the entire time, we spoke little during this early phase. Neither one of us wanted to scare the other, both overwhelmed by the heaviness of the moment. I snapped a few pictures of him staring out the window. These are some of my favorite photos of him. It breaks my heart to know I filled him with so much worry. I often look at these pictures to remind myself just how much this man loves me.

An hour later, I was relieved when I realized that no catastrophic side effects had happened with the Leucovorin. In fact, was it possible that I still felt nothing from the drug? So far, so good…

"Chemo check!"

Enter Oxaliplatin. It was immediately clear that this drug would not be as benign as Leucovorin. Almost as soon as it began flowing through the line, I felt my energy dialing down, my eyelids becoming heavy and my desire to stay engaged in minor conversations dissolving. When I stood up to walk to the bathroom, the room spun away from me. It felt cheeky to ask

Louis to go with me and then refuse to take his arm when he offered it. The IV tree seemed more stable. But I received a static shock when I touched it; it felt like scalding hot ice cubes. This was the cold sensitivity that Terry had warned me about. I had the impression that this side effect appeared days or weeks down the line, not minutes. Oxaliplatin meant business, going to work on me right away.

The bathroom felt like electricity. Everything I touched gave my hands a *zing!* Louis had to touch everything for me. He had to open the door for me, put down the toilet seat and cover it with paper. The grab bar was too cold, so he steadied me as I lowered down on to the freezing seat. The tepid water from the automatic sink was unbearable. I tried using hand sanitizer instead, but the evaporating alcohol gel was icy knives. We tried to wipe it off with a paper towel, but by then I was nearly in tears. I was running out of energy to stand, and I needed some to make it back to my cubicle. I had a brief thought that I might have to stay in the bathroom for the rest of the day.

This was no longer theoretical. Chemotherapy was real, and its effects were tangible. Finally settled back into my reclining chair, I pulled the thin hospital blanket over me. I felt sorry for myself. I wanted to shut my eyes and make the world go away. *Please, everyone, just leave me alone. I don't want to play this game anymore.*

The final two drugs of the day drove the point home. Irinotecan came first. Within minutes, it rendered my mouth almost unusable; speaking was a major effort as I could not enunciate certain letters (L) and letter combinations (words that begin with s-t-r). I panicked, convinced I was having a stroke. Terry did her best to calm me down and reassure me that this side effect would soon pass. Before the next drug arrived, I would have some time to acclimate to my new way of speaking.

As the weeks went on and we knew to expect this side effect, we had fun with it. We amused ourselves by making up tongue twisters for me to say with my fat tongue. Laughter holding our anxieties at bay. It would only last for the 90 minutes that I was getting the Irinotecan, so we learned to hone our craft on a deadline.

The last drug, 5-Fluorouracil (5-FU), was administered in two parts. After being detached from my IV tree, the first part of the dose was administered through what is called a *push*. Terry gave me the first 600mg of the drug with a syringe, slowly pushing the liquid through the primary line left hanging from my portacath. The rest of the 5-FU would be delivered slowly through a small portable pump attached to my portacath. I would bring the little machine home with me for the next 46 hours to finish the infusion. That meant, two days later, Friday afternoon, I would have to return to have it removed. By the end of the day, they had pumped me with nine drugs (four chemotherapy and five supportive).

Seven hours after they administered the first drug, I settled into my bed at home. Without the excitement and distractions of the infusion ward, I was forced to face the chemotherapy head-on. I was not feeling well. I was not hungry. I was tired, sad, frightened, and overwhelmed. I wanted to hide from the drugs, from the cancer and from the world. Louis settled on the bed with me to watch episodes of *X-Files* and offered to bring me whatever I needed so I could stay in bed the rest of the day.

We had to find a way to manage the pump and the long IV line in the bed. It was constantly tugging on my portacath or getting tangled in the blankets. Obviously, men had designed the port: no matter what bra I wore, it would rub on it and bend the IV lines. The dogs both spent time with me on the bed, heads tilted and ears perked with mild curiosity each time the pump's servos kicked on. They would spend the next 46 hours glued to my side: Luna on the bed, pressing herself tight up against me like a puppy; her head resting on my hip; her dark soulful eyes never leaving my face; Dusty curled up on his dog bed on the floor below me. They were my devoted friends, supporting me through these tough days with the pump. Wherever I went in the house, they never left my side. They would repeat this behavior with each subsequent infusion.

Terry had advised me to drink two liters of water while I had the pump attached to me. I had every intention of following her instructions. But my first sip of tepid water was a sip of broken glass. How would I drink *enough* water if I could not drink *any* water? Louis warmed up the teakettle and added hot water to my bottle. He also brought me a small bowl of instant mashed potatoes with butter. I was not hungry. For 20 minutes, I played with those potatoes like the little brother from *A Christmas Story*; I refused to eat them. Appetite loss would get worse over the next two days, and Louis' panic would grow exponentially.

That night, I found it impossible to sleep. I would not skimp on using marijuana during chemo to soothe my insomnia caused by the steroids and adrenalin. Having the pump with me in the bed made me uneasy. Although I slept very little that night, at least the pot brought some calmness, allowing me to settle enough so that Louis could sleep.

The next day, I had even less appetite. Around lunchtime, Louis offered some banana slices, which I stared at for 10 minutes before asking him to take them away. He was pleading with me to eat. No force in the universe was going to compel me to put food in my mouth. I was unmoved by the sight of Louis' desperation. I would lose three of my four precious new pounds with this first infusion.

We returned to the cancer center Friday afternoon to have the pump removed. When they pulled the needle from my portacath, in an instant, I felt the weight lifted off my shoulders. It was difficult knowing I had to go through this process five more times; my head stuck in a downward spiral. On our way home, we were maybe one mile from the cancer center when my complaining began. "I can't believe I have to do this again." The sound of the 5-FU pump's servos had followed me around for three days, like a robotic underscore to my every breath, and now their memory punctuated my complaint.

"You don't have to do it for 10 more days. Let's not worry about that now," Louis soothed. It could have been so easy to waste energy building up stress ahead of the next infusion. My job was to rest and eat as much as possible and try to get back to a sense of normalcy. It was simple math: of the 84 days of chemo, only 18 would be active infusions.

I could do this.

My mood had taken a dark turn during that first infusion, but without the pump hanging off me, I could rise out of my stupor. Over the next few days, the steroids dissipated so I could get some actual sleep. Deep, delicious, bottom-of-the-ocean sleep teeming with strange and vivid dreams.

With each subsequent infusion, we learned to relax more while I rode the wave of side effects. No amount of worry would cure them. A big lesson toward accepting the cone, and not focusing on a potential future reprieve.

Once I got past the first infusion, just as Terry had promised, I became an expert in all things related to FOLFIRINOX, or as we liked to call it, *Folfiritron*. I knew the names of the drugs and the order I got them. I reminded the nurses to add the antibiotic ring to the needle before piercing my port. I scaled back the contents of my supply bag (including downloading the *Harry Potter* books into my iPad so I did not have to waste bag space on heavy hardcovers) and discovered that I needed to pack a snack for myself, too.

Despite all the uncertainty and stress, one thing was clear after my first infusion: I could do this thing with my husband, my son, and my dogs supporting me through the difficult moments and creating an atmosphere at home that was about as normal as possible. With my head in a good place to support my body, the little voice of my spirit could sing the most important song of all:

I am going to live.

FOREIGN BODIES

Following my diagnosis, we purchased a handful of *What to Expect When You're Expecting* type books about chemo and colon cancer. Reluctantly selecting the thinnest book in the stack, I cracked it open and read precisely 100 words before closing it again. I gathered up all the new arrivals and tossed them into the growing heap of books that I never intended to read.

It can be useful to have some idea of what to expect with chemo. But no book could have prepared me for what was going to happen to *me*. I could have consumed all the information available, and it would have made no difference. The moment the first drug dripped into my vein, I would have forgotten all of it. Clearly, knowing everything and knowing nothing were the same thing with chemotherapy. Ultimately, I offered my body to the drugs willingly, unencumbered by any expectations.

I was silent about my health struggles leading up to my diagnosis. Only three people outside of our immediate household knew what was going on. I had not even told my parents what was happening until after I had the first CT scan. Even though I am not a celebrity, I had to think long and hard about a public announcement. I did not need a trickle of information hitting the airwaves, causing people to worry even more because they had to fill in the gaps. I needed to control the message and the situation so that I could convey the information to the most people at once. The last thing I needed was to keep repeating myself while I navigated these whitewater rapids.

I thought long and hard about how to announce, "I have colon cancer." I wanted it to strike as intended: a surprise to everyone. I decided to start a new blog before saying anything on my social media.

What I could not control was how people reacted to the news. Sadly, Nurse Negative Nancy was not the only insensitive person out there waiting for me. Facebook turned out to be a minefield. I stepped on one when someone wrote, "My aunt died of colon cancer. I hope you do better." Other than that, most everyone was sympathetic. Many jumped to action, "I know I live 1000 miles away, but please let me know if there is any way I can help you."

"Please, *please* let me take care of you," my friend Phyllis implored, on the verge of tears, standing on my front porch. Her plea (and subsequent weekly deliveries of homemade root vegetable soups) was my first lesson in how important it is to accept help. It can be just as important for the other person who gives it.

Hearing stories of mundane daily life in a text, receiving weekly humorous greeting cards with a friend's handwriting on them, and opening an unexpected package to find a survivor angel made all the difference in the world. I loved getting random messages and emails. I enjoyed reading the comments readers made on my blog. The countless private messages and gifts I received from people I have known since kindergarten touched me.

The energy everyone put into me was palpable. Sometimes I could *feel* the weight of everyone's energy pressing in on me. It felt as if the world was holding its breath, waiting to hear that I had survived another day. It was magic.

A friend apologized for praying for me. He knows I do not share his beliefs, but he did it because it was something that comforted him. I told him that anyone who focused their positive energy on me was doing a wonderful service. I do not care if it is prayers or meditations or just time spent thinking about me while folding laundry. It was all worthwhile and helpful. Knowing people were sending me positivity was a precious gift.

For a few people, disappearing was the only way they could cope. I struggled with this because it cut deep; I felt abandoned and disillusioned. It would have been nice for them to be a part of this experience, but it was not their path. I had to learn to make peace with their absence. I hoped to find a way to not be weird to them when this was over.

Many people unintentionally projected their worries, fears, and stereotypes on me. Some tried to relate — unsuccessfully, of course — to what I was going through. They could not see that their fears were not my fears. To inject those foreign bodies into my delicate mental state was insensitive, and expectations about my reactions to their feelings felt cruel. I had to be thoughtful about with whom I wanted to interact and how much information I wanted to provide. Overall, people listened patiently, offering an ear and a shoulder with no strings attached. Those who placed no expectations on me gave me the room I needed to tell my story.

What I was not expecting was how people were immediately laser-focused on chemo instead of addressing or acknowledging the cancer itself. Ahead of my first chemo treatment, I was spending most of my time doing whatever I could to remain calm and prepare myself. Some things I was hearing were quite detrimental. Even if someone thought they were being helpful, they were actually creating more fear for me. I would take one step forward in my preparedness, and they would drag me two steps back. I am sure they did not intend to do so, but it affected me deeply.

Cancer gave me the unexpected gift of patience, or at least my version of patience. Something I am not known for. It would have been easy to fall into a depressed funk and just lay in bed feeling sorry for myself for the entire 12 weeks. I fought through the fatigue and side effects, dragging through my day, accomplishing nothing. My body was screaming for rest. I had to accept that it was ok to do nothing all day. I would learn that the best way to fight cancer was by lying down.

I spent most of my time wrapped in cozy blankets while reading and napping on the patio in the sunny Southern California winter afternoons. I had the blog to blow off steam and work through emotions. Louis and a few of my friends encouraged me to use writing to explore my mental journey, and so I poured myself into journaling. I approached writing the same way I did music and yoga: I set a schedule and stuck to it. When I was feeling anxious or pensive, I would write. When I would have been practicing the cello, my burnt fingers were typing away instead, and my head was clearing itself of emotional burdens.

Writing helped me sort out all the complicated and sticky feelings that went along with having cancer. Everyone focused on chemotherapy; they had questions about my physical health.

But no one asked how *my head* was doing. They correctly sensed that the answers would be too distressing for them to process. Several times, I unloaded my actual feelings on some poor unsuspecting friend who was just asking out of politeness. Thankfully, the blog gave people the ability to read only as much as they wanted. They could skip the parts that made them uncomfortable. It had a more important effect on other cancer patients and survivors who continually wrote to me to say: "You might have been describing me."

No one wants to hear the deepest fears of a cancer patient; it's too much to bear. Though I got a lot of comments from healthy folks thanking me and saying they better understood what friends and family had felt during their cancer treatments.

My close friends reached out and spoke to me the same as always. But the less close I was with someone, the more likely they were to use kid gloves around me. They spoke the word *cancer* carefully or tried to avoid saying it at all costs. I know I have **cancer**; it is not a secret. Saying the word does not give me more cancer. Avoiding saying the name only gives the cancer more power. Like Voldemort.

With a lot of time on my hands during chemotherapy, writing was a release valve letting out the back pressure. I could also identify some deep-seated emotions I did not know existed until I chipped away at the surface. There is an outside expectation placed on us to fixate on anger, fear, mortality, and chemotherapy. I know I am not the only cancer survivor spending my time thinking about people and pets and clouds and mountains and realizing I have not spent enough time on this planet.

One toxic bubble that kept rising to the surface, which I tried (and failed) to tamp down, was wondering if I had missed some signs of the cancer long before I saw the doctor. I had to avoid this path at all costs. To think about it would mean that I might have to admit that I had willfully ignored the obvious signs months earlier. Or might prove that I was just like so many women who ignored clear signs of ovarian cancer because it embarrassed them to talk to their doctor. Did I miss something obvious that could have driven me to the doctor a couple of months earlier? Did I bring this on myself?

I had no reason to question my good health. At my annual physical in February 2021, I was healthy. The bloodwork looked great. EKG was normal. All systems go. Mission Control had approved me for my 47th orbit around the sun. Go flight!

HARD THINGS

While hiking, I come across hills of varying grades and technical difficulties. Some only require a little extra effort. Other inclines require me to dig deep for the endurance to manage a long climb of a mile or more. Going up one of the more difficult hills, I keep my mind focused on the place where I am and my goal of reaching the top. It is my nature to avoid lifting my eyes to see the top of the trail, my gaze fixed just a few feet ahead of where I am stepping. I never worry about how I will get back down the trail or how many more hills might wait on the other side. I am too busy working out where to place my next step. Since there are no piles of human skeletons littering the trail, I feel pretty confident that everyone makes it back alive.

After my cancer diagnosis, I realized that this had all been a dress rehearsal for chemotherapy. Keeping my mind on where I am and what I am doing, and not looking too far ahead into the future, proved essential with chemo. Thinking a couple of weeks or months into the future would have driven me crazy. It was essential that Louis reminded me to keep my mind on the treatment I was going through, to stay in the present, and not worry about potential additional treatments in the coming months. No reason to worry about the possibility of radiation. I needed to get through chemo. No reason to worry about the next surgery while I was trying to survive radiation. I needed a lot of reminders and support from Louis to keep me thinking that way, but in the end, it was worth the effort and energy.

As soon as my chemotherapy ended, I gave myself permission to research all the information on the drugs that I had been avoiding, curious to see if I had had the expected side effects. I wanted to learn more about the drugs themselves. Among the piles of information, I found out that I received the 5-FU above the average dosage. It would have been a terrible mind game to play if I had known that while hooked to the pump.

Mouth sores were, by far, the most shocking side effect I suffered. Friends talked about them but did them no justice. These things were no joke. My tongue looked like a piece of chopped meat. Under my tongue was red and swollen, it felt like I was holding gumballs under my tongue all the time. The insides of my cheeks swelled up and broke open. They rubbed against my teeth when I spoke and made it difficult to close my mouth without biting down on them. My gums burned all the time as if I had eaten scalding hot pizza, shredding and peeling the same way. When I brushed my teeth, my gums would bleed. My toothbrush bristles perpetually stained pink. It hurt to speak; it hurt to swallow. It hurt to eat; it hurt to drink. It hurt to shut my mouth; it hurt to open my mouth. I was miserable, and there was nothing I could do about it. A friend told me that during chemo, their mouth sores were so bad they drove to a gun store and sat in the parking lot contemplating suicide. I suffered enough; I cannot imagine what they went through.

My mouth sores would often subside to a more tolerable level between infusions. During that week, I would attempt to eat calorie-rich foods. Unfortunately, my tongue was so damaged that I could not taste much of anything. Not being able to taste made eating highly unpleasant, and in my case, left me disinterested in food altogether. I discovered that sucking on ginger candies before eating could sometimes help cut through the muck. It was imperative that we found foods I could taste through the dead taste buds, so I gravitated toward bold and spicy flavors, which in turn burned my mouth. There was no winning.

One day Louis found me cheerfully eating grapes, not knowing that both he and Andrew had declared them sour and sentenced them to the trash. I tasted nothing. Because the cold sensitivity would wane between treatments, I was enjoying the sensation of the cold juice popping on the sores in my mouth.

Dr. Quilici and Dr. Jacobs cautioned Louis: "None of this will work if she doesn't eat." He took this seriously. Gaining weight was my only responsibility and feeding me was Louis' full-time job. Finding something (anything) that I would eat willingly was our top priority, even if that meant sour grapes.

Chemotherapy drugs kill off fast growing cells. This includes taste buds. Many cancer patients report a *metallic flavor*. I never described that taste that way; I thought it gave the impression of dead or dying tissue. Unable to taste food was bad enough. But to be overwhelmed with this flavor when I had a mouthful of one of the few foods I still enjoyed (like macaroni and cheese) ruining any small enjoyment I was getting felt like a cruel joke. I came away from this side effect disgusted by peppers, mushrooms, onions, sage, oregano, certain vegan meats, and a bunch of other healthy and normally delicious foods.

Because the flavor would creep up on me with no warning, I carried sugar-free ginger candies with me everywhere I went.

It helped to mask the flavor, but I just had to be patient and wait for this to pass. It took about seven months for it to stop happening, but by then I was already avoiding a lot of foods I had previously enjoyed. My post-chemo diet was bland, but slowly it would come back over the following year.

Adding to the problem was the cold sensitivity caused by the Oxaliplatin. This meant for the first week of each infusion, I could not eat the cold foods which I could have used to soothe the mouth wounds (this ruled out my favorite calorie-dense protein shakes). On the rare occasions when I was genuinely hungry, there were few foods I could tolerate inside my mouth. I lived on soft mushy foods, like mashed potatoes and macaroni and cheese, which Louis would cool by blowing on, as for a toddler.

Cold sensitivity ruled my life. It is difficult to convey the experience. This was nothing like feeling fever chills or having teeth that are sensitive to ice cream. The sensation was jarring and sometimes frightening. Deeply rooted in the nerves themselves, the sensations bordered on knifelike pain. Touching something cool felt like touching a hot stove burner. Every nerve ending screamed, making it impossible to decipher if what I was touching was hot or cold.

During the 5-FU infusions, my hands would cramp and gnarl into inhuman shapes, and I lost feeling in them. This was the scary side effect, neuropathy, that everyone had hoped this musician would avoid. Would my hands ever unfurl again? On the verge of hysteria, the more I panicked, the more they curled, Louis trying everything he could to calm me down. Because it continued to happen multiple times per day, I figured out that a severe cold sensitivity reaction almost always triggered these spasms. I learned that wearing light gloves all day, sleeping with them on at night, and either sitting on my hands or keeping them in my armpits could stave this off, mostly.

With my bald head and disposable white cotton gloves on, Louis said one night as we watched tv in bed, "I feel like I'm cuddling with the butler."

Even with the gloves on all the time, I was reflexively throwing things down. Often, I forgot myself and picked up something cool, like a fork, or tried to handle the frozen soups that Andrew was bringing home for me. Neuropathy persisted for over a year. I wondered if I would ever feel any relief from this side effect. It was ok to ask for help. Otherwise, all the food in the freezer would end up on the floor.

My feet were the same. The terrazzo and hardwood floors were intolerable to my bare feet. Mirroring what I was experiencing in my hands, my feet cramped into their own unique versions of fists, which made it difficult to walk or stay balanced. Now I understood why we were told to be aware of tripping hazards in our house. I never walked around barefoot, always wearing shoes, hard-soled slippers, or thick grippy socks. Getting out of the shower, I would jump between bathmats to avoid stepping on the cold bathroom tiles like I was playing the childhood lava game.

The cold sensitivity extended to my mouth and throat, as well. Brushing my teeth with peppermint toothpaste and cool water would make my tongue curl and my steroid moon-face twist into horrifying masks. In any other situation, that might be amusing. But this was one of the more frightening sights I saw in the mirror. I switched to children's watermelon-flavored toothpaste and warm water.

Louis, the constant observer of my every waking moment, had to come to grips with my wild energy swings and appetite issues. He was beside himself with worry during my first infusion, when I was fighting oppressive fatigue. He wondered if it might be depression setting in. Every instinct was screaming to make me do things. Eventually, he accepted that there would be times I might not get up off the bed or sofa, no matter what he did. Over time, he came to understand the patterns of each infusion. He learned how best to support and help me through it. If Louis stayed relaxed, I might relax as well.

"What's your chemo-craving?" Amanda, my friend who is a cancer survivor, texted me one evening during my third infusion. "I was obsessed with chocolate croissants," she proclaimed. Suddenly, chocolate croissants were my obsession, too.

"Meatballs. All I want is meatballs..." not realizing this was because of chemo. I made myself some amazing vegan meatball subs at home and added meatless meatballs to everything I ate. At one point, I just heated a pot of tomato sauce, threw in some meatballs, and ate the whole thing with a wooden spoon. It did not matter how much my mouth burned from the acidity; I could not get enough of them. Tragically, after chemo, I could not stand the sight or smell of those once beloved meatballs.

Just when we thought we had a handle on the appetite, fatigue, cold sensitivity, mouth sores, and all the other major side effects, it horrified us to watch as the skin started peeling from my hands. Until this point, I only had dry skin and a slight pink tint to my palms; I did not appreciate why Dr. Jacobs was making such a fuss about inspecting my hands at my weekly appointments. Even though I did not understand what his motives were, I took his advice and kept them slathered in cream under my gloves. I remained blissfully unaware of how serious Hand and Foot Syndrome, caused by the 5-FU, would be.

Halfway through my treatments, every crease and line in my palms became red and burnt and cracked open, and the skin peeled away in strips between my fingers. The webbing between my thumb and forefinger was a painful, open wound for countless weeks. The precious calluses that string players rely on were lifting off like little skin buttons, and it was painful to play my cello. My cuticles cracked and bled, my nails lifted off the nail beds and receded. I was lucky that the drugs spared my feet this torture.

More than once, Dr. Jacobs took my disintegrating hands tenderly in his and condoled, "You poor thing."

Week after week, he would reassure me that all would heal after chemo ended. I was one of the most severe cases of Hand and Foot Syndrome he had ever seen. I just had to remember, "This is all temporary."

Chemotherapy stands like a towering mountain peak, dreamlike, poking through the clouds that surround my cancer treatments. Trying to remember what chemo was like plays like a movie I saw long ago as a child or a story someone read to me while I was drifting off to sleep. I cannot believe it was *me* that did this incredible and difficult thing.

"*I can do hard things,*" Lori's voice echoed in my head. This qualified.

It is impossible to feel *normal* during chemo, though many of us use that word in a lame attempt to describe what we do to cope during treatments. Some people go to work or raise small children while on chemo. Even then, it can hardly be called *normal*. It is just something that must be done. I was incapable of doing anything meaningful. I was a useless blob, often unable and unwilling to answer my phone. Speaking took so much energy. Most of the time I was so deep in my protective cocoon

I was unwilling to engage in the simple act of moving my mouth and forming words.

Friends who came to see me during chemo were shocked by how devastated my body was. That was my fault. I took great care to take photos of myself doing yoga or out hiking with the dogs, exuding resilience and positivity. But it was all white lies and tricks of the camera. I only practiced yoga through the first four infusions. After that, I struggled to hold myself up long enough to get to the bathroom; but I posted old photos, pretending I was still on the mat. Hiking became a nightmare. Even on the flats, I got winded and needed to stop to catch my breath. If I made it to the top of a hill, I would lean on my trekking poles and cry while Louis reassured me it was just a byproduct of the chemo doing its job. After I settled down, he would snap a photo. Of course, to the rest of the world, it looked like I was doing great.

Getting through chemotherapy was *hard work* every single day. My struggle was just as much about the head games as the physical discipline. I tried desperately to keep things under control. The worst emotions did not even have names attached to them. Crying became my language of choice when I could not muster the energy to just get my socks on. Internal dialogue was no longer possible; I just had buckets of emotional overload spilling out of me. It was almost as if there was a second, crazy version of Lisa traveling along inside of me. There was no controlling her. These were her outbursts punctuating my day unexpectedly.

There were more times than I can count when tears would flow for no reason. We would watch tv and without warning, I would weep uncontrollably. At the slightest inconvenience in the kitchen, I would scream at Louis at the top of my lungs. I would sit on the chair in our closet in my underwear and cry until he found me and helped me get dressed. We learned to live with the outbursts. We both had to accept that there was no fixing whatever it was I was feeling. He only had to help me get through it.

I'm just so tired, was an unintended mantra. Sometimes I said it like this was a surprise. Other times I would say it like I was ready to lie down and die. I knew the fatigue would increase until the final infusion, when Dr. Jacobs promised it would be almost intolerable, and yet I could not wrap my brain around the reality of it. "I'm just so tired," I would moan, and Louis could only respond, "I know you are."

I had no choice. I would never walk into Dr. Jacobs' office the morning of an infusion and say, "No thanks. Not today. I'm done with this." With stage-4 cancer, the only choices I had were to live or die. There was no middle ground. My determination to complete my treatments helped me find the strength to make it through all six doses. My desire to live was overwhelming. I felt it in every cell in my body. I would finish treatments with no delays even if it killed me.

Chemotherapy damages the bone marrow. I knew this in theory and experienced it firsthand. Every week, my blood tests confirmed what physical exertion had already illustrated for me: my red blood cell count was low, I was anemic. Even more worrisome for me, Dr. Jacobs, and the nurses at the infusion center was that my white blood cell count was even lower. With the coronavirus pandemic still raging outside our home, we were doing everything we could to keep me safe from infections. After my third treatment, Dr. Jacobs had to decide if I would receive the next three infusions on time because my white cell count was on the borderline of being too low to allow me to receive my drugs.

The thought of skipping, postponing, or ending the treatments scared me. The only way I knew to live was with the drugs. They kept the cancer from taking over my body, but they also kept it from taking over my mind. The drugs had become my security blanket. There was no stopping now. "If your numbers get worse, we may have to postpone for a week," Dr. Jacobs informed me. An icy chill filled me.

No. I don't like this idea at all.

There is no magical way to regrow white blood cells in a week. I had hoped I would be the one person to discover the secret. The only thing I could do was turn all my energies toward willing my bone marrow to heal itself, because no way was I going to miss or postpone treatment. Not now. This train was barreling down the track, and I was not going to let anything stop it. I honestly do not know how it happened, but when I arrived at the office for my fourth infusion, my white blood cell count had not continued to drop. In fact, it had gone up two-tenths from 1.4 to 1.6. Good enough! Bring on the next infusion.

This is how I continued for three more infusions: head down, eyes straight ahead, grow some fresh blood, and hit me again. I did the hard thing six times, which was five more times than I expected. I have a residual mix of pride and disbelief in myself for being able to complete all six treatments.

By the end of those 12 weeks, my exhaustion was on full display. I had a heavy way of walking with a hitching limp. My lash-less eyelids were pink, swollen, heavy, and crusty all the time. My mouth was numb and chewed up. I had exactly two hundred strands of grey hair on my head, and my hands looked like I had dipped them in acid; crochet beanies and white gloves had taken over an entire drawer in my dresser. I had difficulty swallowing, and I had acid reflux. My nose was running constantly and in the mornings, it bled. I sounded like I had a perpetual head cold. My ears rang, and my eyesight was getting worse. And yet, I would make myself repeat, "Chemo is my friend and ally and my most powerful weapon against cancer." This constant reminder redirected my frustration where it belonged: on the cancer, not on the chemo. I needed every ounce of courage to get through the treatment.

I doubt I will ever recover from the heavy emotional weight of the drugs being pumped into me. The sound of the portable pump replayed in my head long after chemotherapy ended. In the middle of the night, when everything else is silent, I still hear the servos burst into action. Like so many other survivors before me, this aural trauma will leave a deep echo in my soul; I expect the sound of those servos will haunt me for the rest of my life.

The Poison Cure.

We can do incredible things when our lives are on the line.

I missed being me. Not only because of the stranger in the mirror, but because my daily routine was gone. I was no longer a person I recognized. I would moan my frustrations to Louis while I stood in the door to my yoga-slash-music room, staring longingly at my cellos. Chemo was saving my life, but stripping away the things that made me, *me*. It would not always be like this. But at my lowest, *someday soon* might as well have been a lifetime away.

I avoided making eye contact with my bald and swollen face in the mirror. I felt out of control. The assortment of gadgets and gizmos hanging off my body had transformed me into an alien robot.

Everything sucked. It all sucked big time.

The drugs are there to destroy cancer. But in that process, they destroy our body and our sense of normalcy. The side effects are powerful. So sometimes it felt like it was all I could do to hold myself together against the onslaught. Instead of resenting the outward effects of the drugs, I would remind myself that the tumor was suffering much worse. My mouth was filled with sores, the tumor was burning. My hair was falling out, the shell of the tumor was being breached. My bone marrow was dying, the center of the tumor was dissolving. That was key: visualizing the cancer cells dissolving into nothing, just like my dream showed me, and just as Dr. Jacobs had divined. Thinking about this made it easier to cope with the side effects. They were a necessary reality.

What I really needed was some sleep. So while I laid in bed, the pump's servos springing to life every 90 seconds, administering another dose of the 5-FU, I would think, *Take that, cancer. Eff you.*

LUCKY

One Friday, as we returned to the infusion center to have my pump removed, we came across an old woman in the parking garage: holding on to her daughter's arm, stooped and shuffling, wearing a coat and hat too heavy for a beautiful February day in Southern California.

"That's what chemo actually looks like." Louis directed my attention to her. "*Now,* do you understand why everyone's so pleased with how well you're doing?"

He was right. Walking through the infusion center or the oncology office, the nurses always said to me, "You look great!" Several times, Dr. Jacobs told me outright how pleased he was with how well I was tolerating the drugs. Some weeks, I walked into appointments nearly normal — feeling energetic, talking about what I was going to eat for lunch, showing off my bald head, and making *dad jokes* about my colostomy.

I was so lucky.

Observing the other patients in the infusion center, I saw people who shuffled in, leaning on walkers, pushed in wheelchairs, grasping canes, hanging desperately onto their companions, hunched over, shaking, shriveled, and beaten down. I walked in and out of all six infusions of my own power.

I was so lucky.

There are people who cannot afford good health insurance. People who cannot take time off from work while they go through chemo. People who cannot pay their medical bills. And here I am at the Disney Family Cancer Center, one of the best hospitals in one of the largest cities in the world, paired up with two of the best oncologists and surgeons in Los Angeles, and an insurance company that has covered my medical bills exceeding one million dollars without question.

I was so lucky.

Countless friends held us up, tending to our every need. Louis and our boys did not have to worry about anything except helping me get through this. My son and stepsons are thriving and healthy, and my husband loves me.

I am so lucky.

HAIR TODAY, GONE TOMORROW

Two of the most common anxieties anyone has ahead of chemotherapy are: will I be sick, and will I lose my hair?

We have all seen pictures of bald cancer patients. Smooth heads seem to be the requisite look, the hat of the cancer uniform. Every character in a tv show or movie who goes through chemo loses their hair on the first day, dramatic clumps coming out in their fingers. Many take razors and clippers to their scalps to expedite the process (some even give birth to their alter ego). Although pop culture said otherwise, there was no absolute rule that my hair would fall out just because I was having chemotherapy. And even if it did fall out, there was no guarantee I would end up bald.

In the weeks before my chemotherapy began, I did not give hair loss much thought. The more stomach-y side effects of diarrhea, nausea, and vomiting occupied my mind. Being told my hair would thin out felt like a *get-out-of-jail-free* card, so I gave myself permission to ignore the idea completely.

During my first infusion, I noticed that there was more hair caught in my brush than was usual. I was not going to worry about it. But, when my hair started falling out for real, it was accompanied by a healthy dose of denial. Unlike women in the movies, I did not *bravely* rush to shave my head.

The first sign that it was happening occurred during the second infusion. The morning I was to return to the infusion center to have the pump removed, things spiraled rapidly. While I was shampooing, my fingers got tangled in my hair and I had to tug and pull to get them free. I drew back my hands to find great clumps of hair wrapped around my fingers. This happened multiple times during my shower. The water was backing up in the tub above my ankles. The amount of hair in the drain was astounding. It looked like a cat died at the bottom of the tub. I was mortified. Could this be happening?

By the time I finished that shower, there was hair all over my back, shoulders, and stomach, twisted between my toes, and hanging from my port line to the 5-FU pump. Even without my glasses on and steam covering the mirror, I could see that a wide bald line of skin now snaked its way along my skull from my forehead to my nape. It was obvious what was happening. But I could not admit what was so clear in front of my blurry eyes.

My hair was supposed to *thin out*. This seemed like more than that. My appointment to have the 5-FU pump removed that afternoon loomed dark. At least I could ask the nurses about my hair situation and see what they thought. If there was a way out of this puzzle, an obvious solution, they would give me the key.

Abby, another of my nurses at the infusion center, is a joyful, positive, plain-spoken shining light of a woman whose spirit seems impervious to all the cancer surrounding her. When we arrived that afternoon, I showed her the bald spots and thick bare line on the top of my head. She said it looked like I was going to lose all my hair. Prepare myself for it. She reminded me that many women shave their heads when they reach the point I was at, which helped them feel as if they still had some control over the situation.

While she was talking, the defiant inner voice of Stubborn Lisa spoke up: "Doesn't matter, I'm not going to lose my hair." I replaced the knit hat on my head. Out of sight, out of mind, right? I convinced myself that by thrusting my head into the sand, I could will my remaining hair to stick to my scalp. What if I pinched my nose and held my breath? Would new hairs sprout?

The evening crawled on. I spent most of it rationalizing and contemplating the situation. None of this felt good. I was not afraid of being bald or shaving my head. What I feared was that I would jump the gun and shave my head before knowing for certain all my hair was going to fall out. What if this was all the hair I was going to lose? Shaving my head would seem pointless and presumptive. I would have made myself bald for no good reason.

All I knew was that shaving would mean the cancer was real. I cannot keep up the façade without my hair.

I was being dragged down by the hair clinging to the back of my shirt. I was afraid to touch my head because every time I did, I came back with clumps of hair sticking to my peeling palms. I felt the weight of my ego bearing down on my shoulders. Turns out, I was quite vain about my thick auburn hair with the grey streaks at my temples.

My friend Amanda has the most beautiful hair I have ever seen in real life. Her naturally curled Superman black hair seems to shine with a blue glow. It always left me aching with envy. She would be a pillar of support for me through the hair phase of my chemo.

I texted her that night to ask how she coped with her hair loss. I expected something more emotional than what she had told me. Her hair started falling out in the morning and that same afternoon she shaved her head. She sent me her before-and-after photos, taken just hours apart. She was beautiful with her fabulous hair, but it was nothing compared to how gorgeous she was with a shaved head. I was stunned by the photos: in the *before* photo, she looked dark and uncertain; in the *after* photo, she looked vibrant and unburdened.

Inspired, I decided I wanted to take a *before* picture of myself, too. On any other day, I would have put on an artificial smile, written a "Ha-ha my hair is falling out #fuckcancer" caption, and used a flattering filter to make my life seem a lot shinier than it really was. It took copious amounts of courage to capture reality instead.

The face staring back from the mirror was heavy and troubled. The unintended colors in the photo seemed to match my mood: beige and blah. I texted this photo to my friend Ella, and she responded, "I've never seen that look on your face before and I hope I never see it again. You'll feel better once you shave."

I went to bed that night wondering how I would know it was the right time to shave. Would it come as a lightning bolt, or would it continue as this slow burn?

The next morning, Saturday, I decided some quiet yoga would help. Even though I was feeling fatigue from chemo, I knew getting on the mat was important to coming to terms with this situation. The problem was not finding the energy to do the yoga. The actual problem was getting my hair into a ponytail. Every time I tried to gather my hair together, more strands would fall out in my hands. I would get a rubber band around the hair, but on the final wrap, it would slip out; so much hair was shedding, the elastic had nothing to anchor to. I was no longer feeling sad about my situation. I was feeling annoyed and pissed off. This was an important shift.

I compromised by putting my hair into a bandana, with no ponytail necessary. My yoga practice was short, slow, and gentle. Just enough time to allow me to think about my hair situation. I needed to make a plan. When I finished my practice, Louis came into the room to talk to me about something unrelated to me, cancer, or my hair. I was not having any of that. I only wanted to talk about my hair.

We sat for quite some time, perhaps longer than we should have, talking about the existential effects of shaving. I knew I was at a very important juncture in my life. I cannot grow or move toward a better me by hanging on to my old decorations.

Now, several years in remission, Amanda's hair is back and as beautiful as ever. She told me that part of the healing process after cancer was watching her hair grow back, an unmistakable sign that her body was clearing the drugs. Ella said that her straight blond hair grew back curly and brown, and 10 years later, she still celebrates her recovery by letting her hair continue to grow long over the years.

My mind made up, I popped off the mat. "Let's go do this thing!" I raced to the bathroom to get the clippers, Louis hot on my heels. Bursting with energy and the thrill of doing something that, on any other day, would be crazy. I had a genuine opportunity to shave my head and see what that was like. Not every woman gets this opportunity, cancer or no cancer. I counted myself lucky to have this experience.

Working together, we pulled my remaining hair into the best ponytail we could manage. With the scissors, Louis started cutting above the rubber band. At that moment, feeling the release of that heavy tail coming off, my spirits rose. As a thoughtful gesture, Louis put the ponytail away for me. It would be a memento of my former life that I would use over the next year to compare the difference in color as my hair grew back.

Louis went back to work, enthusiastically cutting big chunks of hair away. I now sported a cool hairdo, which would have made my 1980s teenage self jealous. After snapping a few photos and making a comment about how *mint* my hair looked, Louis turned on the clippers.

That sound, that heavy click as it burst into life, lives loud in my memory. I had never shaved my head before; this was all new and thrilling. As he ran the clippers over and over and over my skull, I was positively giddy! He handed me the clippers so I could take a few passes at it myself.

The only word to describe this experience was *liberating*. Never have I felt such an immediate and obvious change in attitude. Fluffy, soft chunks of hair fluttered to the floor around my feet, but it felt like lead weights were being thrown off my chest and shoulders. And then it was done. I laughed. I looked like my father. We went out to the patio and Louis snapped pictures of me smiling in the sunshine.

I had been a chrysalis. I shed my shell, my hair, so I could become a butterfly. The change in my attitude was not subtle. I looked like me again. Cancer? Not a trace of it in my smile.

•　　•　　•　　•　　•

If hair holds trauma, and cancer is trauma, then cutting my hair would represent release. Instinctually, we view people with bare heads as delicate, and in need of compassion, baldness an outward sign that someone is healing or ailing, and a call for others to practice compassion and assist in their care. The military buzzes all heads to promote the equality of everyone on the team. And in some religions, hair represents the last vestige of ego. Shaving represents the shedding of vanity in favor of humility and giving oneself over to the path of enlightenment. My mind seemed to embrace all four concepts simultaneously.

The powerful camaraderie among cancer patients was palpable each time I walked into the cancer center sporting my bald head. We are a team; we are one, and we are fighting this battle together, even if we have to do it alone.

The trauma part interests me quite a bit. I have lived an interesting life, and despite my outward positive attitude, it has been tough at times. Someone once told me, "Don't rush to judge, because you never know the path someone has traveled." My path has been winding and often covered in thick brambles. Sure, I have had traumas in my life (who has not had bad things happen to them?), but I have little to complain about. Or at least I thought that before I shaved my head. Perhaps the traumas did not need to be examined by my conscious mind; I only needed to clear the path and allow my unconscious self to release them. Each strand on the floor represented another unnamed trauma that I was letting go.

Everyone suffers from vanity to some degree. Until I had to say goodbye to my hair, I thought I was mostly free from that particular flaw. I never walked around thinking *I'm beautiful,* or *I hope others like the way I look.* I have never measured my attractiveness against the length of my hair. I let the grey grow in naturally and most days wore my hair in a ponytail. But when faced with letting it go, I struggled mightily.

The comments I received when I posted my *after* photos on the blog surprised me. Many of the commenters assumed the loss of my hair left me questioning my self-worth. I got several comments with the same underlying theme: "It's ok, you *still* look beautiful!" "It doesn't matter, you *still* look amazing!" "Don't worry, you *still* look great!"

It sounds a little egotistical, and ironic, to react: I know I'm *still* beautiful. That was never in question. It was interesting how people assumed I was questioning my beauty now that I had no hair. I thought my attitude about my appearance in the past would have already shown that I cared little about these sorts of things. I had made no comments on my photos hinting that I was upset about my hair being gone, either. In fact, the caption I had attached to the photos was: "Feeling like me again."

This feedback set me on an exploration of my stubborn reaction to the situation. I had taken a full spin off in the opposite direction, landing firmly in the Pride camp instead. It pleased me to know that when people saw me, there would be no mistaking I had cancer. I was fighting for my life. If I was going to go through all these treatments, then I would get the acknowledgment I craved from strangers. I got that validation when an old man winked at me in the waiting room while I waited for a PET scan.

It took two weeks for the rest of my hair to fall off my head. The short strands made less of a mess on my pillow and in the shower drain as they continued to fall out. By the 4th infusion, all my body hair was gone as well. I was relieved that my eyebrows remained. Losing my eyelashes hit me the hardest of all. Without lashes, I had several eye problems to contend with, which made it uncomfortable to wear my contact lenses. A friend sent some fake eyelashes, which helped me strike up a cautious relationship with my reflection. Hiding my eyes behind my glasses also helped.

After acclimating to my new look, it amused me to discover that I enjoyed having a shaved head. I loved feeling the breeze blowing through the short hairs. I loved running my hands over the stubble and feeling the ridges and canyons of my skull. My life was instantly simplified. I loved being able to do yoga without hair getting in my face. I loved playing my cello without my hair tangling in the tuning pegs. Showers took less time without having to shampoo and condition long hair. I wondered if I would want to grow my hair back right away. Maybe I would end up wanting to keep the shaved head look for a while.

The emotions I grappled with leading up to the shave were more complicated and yet simpler than anyone outside could grasp. Because none of those contemplations were about my appearance. It ultimately boiled down to one powerful revulsion: I did not want to see a cancer patient in the mirror.

MODERN DAY MONSTER

Having cancer in 2022 meant I had a very public struggle ahead of me. It made no difference if I *wanted* to share. This was the reality of living in this era. People share everything on social media. I could either fight it or accept it, but the decision was mine to allow my cage match with cancer to be filmed before a live studio audience.

I found it very difficult to keep the diagnosis process a secret and away from social media. Not because I was holding back and eager to share, but because one ominous little slip might have triggered people. "What's going on?" I wanted control over when and how I announced my news to the world.

I interacted with people less as I was going through the tests before my diagnosis. But people are not stupid. I could not control how weight loss and low energy appeared in person. Other musicians at rehearsals and concerts could see it. I was surrounded by sensitive people who reached out on a hunch, offering unsolicited and unexpected relief. They may not have known what that support was for, but they were deep wells of strength during those tough months. Without them, it may not have been possible to get through that period of my life in one piece. Pam and Ella knew the full story. They were watching my decline unfold in real time. But Lori, being in New York, only saw the images I wanted her to see. I thought I was sparing her from worry by controlling the message. But I think it made things worse for her when the diagnosis finally came down.

Regardless of the outside pressure to perform, I had to decide if I wanted to share this experience on social media. Was this something that I wanted to commit to doing? I was not going to not create *First Day of School* posts with little chalkboards announcing the start of each chemo treatment. If I gave away the tiniest detail, even if by accident, then the expectation to see photos and blog updates along the way would always be there. There also existed the outside possibility that if people found out that I had been dealing with cancer for months without their knowing, *they* might take offense or have their feelings hurt. As strange as it sounds, I wanted to avoid future resentments, even if just for the selfish reason of preserving my future sanity.

Initially created with the best intentions, my blog could become an uncontrollable Frankensteinian monster unless I set some boundaries. Week after week, I was writing about my internal turmoil; my readers became deeply invested in my progress and often asked for more frequent updates. When I was feeling my shittiest, posting shiny photos or writing a quippy essay about how well things appeared to be going was the last thing I wanted to do. Though I usually gave in to the pressure and wrote updates when I least felt like it, I discovered safety in hiding behind the written word. This allowed me to create whatever reality I wanted to present to my audience. I learned how to construct a world in which I could function in a glass bowl within a lead-lined cask.

In contrast to the coziness afforded by the blog, the expectations of a social media post centered on me putting on a floor show for the audience. Though they may not have realized it, viewers got comfort from seeing photos of me as a thriving cancer patient. Through movies and television, we are shown the stereotypical images of people suffering from cancer. But in real life, people crave alternative images. Everyone is desperate to know their friend's cancer is not as frightening as it looks in those commercials. Since most of the people I connect with on Facebook do not live close enough to witness my daily struggles, these posts gave me an opportunity to soothe everyone's fears by sharing photos of myself looking and acting almost normally through the treatments.

The dark side of that was the expectation of a steady stream of smiling, normal-looking photos. I often felt like I was letting people down if I posted anything hinting at the contrary. When my hair was falling out, I posted an extensive head-shaving collage. It was scary hitting *publish,* but it was also liberating. There was nothing wrong with showing the world how difficult and yet how easy it was to shave my head. And although it was scary to share a set of photos that captured a wide range of emotions that were not all sunny smiles, I had conveyed a deeper meaning to my readers. If I had stuck with the rose color, soft filter lie, I may not have been able to get this point across. People needed to see the crime scene photos with all the gory details.

I had a voice and I was going to use it to say something. It was not up to me to decide if what I was posting was important, interesting, or sane. The reader had to decide what they got out of it. My only duty was to speak from my heart, to be transparent, raw, vulnerable, and fragile. If I put every detail into my story, then it would be clear that I was being completely honest. By not censoring myself, they were more likely to trust me.

I could not avoid posting photos of myself looking positive and somewhat normal because these had the important effect of helping *me* to recover between treatments. Just like my audience, I needed to see photos of normal-looking Lisa to shift my perspective and show myself that I was doing well. In essence, I was inspiring myself. Often when we were hiking in the week between my infusions, I struggled up the steep hills because of my low red blood cell count. Panting and exhausted out of my mind, Louis would stop me. "I need to take a picture of you." I would stop, make a funny face for the camera, and then continue on the trail. Later, when he showed me the pictures, I expected to see a blathering mess, but instead I saw someone who looked mostly alright. It gave me a lot of perspective on the situation and reassured me that my friends were not crazy; they saw what was right in front of their eyes: in the grand scheme of things, I *was* doing ok.

It was impossible to photograph what was going on inside of my brain. Emotional turmoil did not present as a recognizable facial expression for an Instagram post. No camera invented could capture those feelings to make them plain to see. Whatever people saw in the pictures, I hoped they understood the waters ran even deeper.

I used a lot of my blog writing energy trying to dispel the common misconception that cancer patients spend all our time anxious about chemo and contemplating our mortality. Sometimes I thought about it, but I never wrote about it. Those were very private moments, for me and Louis only. Those things I kept to myself were mind-bogglingly complex, at other times embarrassingly pedestrian, but always impossible to explain. Even to my husband.

Separate from my cancer treatments, I wanted to show other ostomates that life does not end just because of a stoma. So, I posted photos and videos of myself doing yoga with my colostomy bag showing. It was just as important for *me* to see those images as it was for them. For the first 4 treatments, that was what I could portray: I feel like crap, and I have this stupid bag, but dammit, I am on my mat!

Every Instagram-ready photo garnered multiple comments like, "You still look beautiful," or "You look great!" Of course I did. I had deliberately crafted the photos to elicit those precise responses. On my blog, I often repeated the complaint: "I don't see myself in the mirror anymore." It had nothing to do with the pictures I posted on social media. It had everything to do with my life behind the scenes. Every day, I watched, helpless, as another piece of my normal life sloughed away before my eyes. Very few people understood this because the pictures were a contradiction.

My little body had been through the wringer. Yet I was hiding the tough images that showed that reality from the public. It took me a while, but I learned the lesson: by posting shiny photos, I did not allow people the chance to fully grasp what was happening to me. I was not getting the support and reactions that I needed because I had single-handedly created the misconception myself.

Multiple times each day, I stood in front of the mirror in my yoga-slash-music room, brazenly engaged in a staring match with the stranger before me. Sometimes I flinched at my reflection and broke down with inconsolable rage at the unfairness of *me* going through this. And other times I dug deep and reassured my reflection, "You're doing really well!" To my eyes, I looked like something out of a sci-fi movie, covered in gadgets, gizmos, servos, access points, release valves, pouches, tubes, and wires. I was rattled by the sight of myself with all that crap attached to me. I had to learn to accept what I saw. My version of *the cone*, which Dr. Jacobs had promised was temporary, only defined this period of my life. It did not define *me*.

Everything fucking sucked. With each passing week, the side effects became harder and harder to cope with and recover from. I consider myself an insightful and observant person, capable of rationalizing myself out of almost any situation. Chemo pushed me to the threshold of what I thought I was capable of and then gave me a hard shove over the cliff. All the physical challenges aside, it took a lot of brainpower to get through this. I discovered I could do some unbelievable things when my life was at stake.

All chemotherapy drugs are *big drugs*. They are scary. They are aggressive. But they were my allies. Humans with the best intentions to save and cure other humans spent decades of their lives devoted to creating these drugs, and all that positive intention was inside the drugs. I just had to be brave enough to be open to that energy.

It was so frightening to know I was going to take these drugs. I had to grapple with both my naïveté and brazen confidence perched on my shoulders and whispering in my ears. There were contradictions in my attitude that I had to face down with honesty and humility. All jammed into sharp focus the moment I felt the needle pierce my port for the first infusion. This experience opened my eyes to the seriousness of setting aside irrational fears and doing what it takes to survive.

Like a clueless rabbit in the yard, Death had been stalking me while I played in the grass. I almost lost. This was no longer theoretical. I only know that every day past my diagnosis was an extra day of life. I read somewhere, by accident of course, since I had been avoiding searching out statistics, that colon cancer has a 5-year survival rate of 10%. Cancer math kicked in: 10 people in line at the store, nine of us would be dead in 5 years. Was Nurse Negative Nancy being generous in her prediction? My life was being divided into tiny 5-year chunks, memories spinning before my eyes like a kaleidoscope. Could I be dead in 2027? Whether or not this is true, I convinced myself that it was the rate for those who did not have treatments. Otherwise, I would go crazy thinking about that statistic. I knew too many people in real life who had survived 10 or more years past their diagnosis of colon cancer, including my great uncles who lived 30 years beyond their cancers. I had to work very hard every day to keep myself from flipping out.

One day, I was hiking on a trail that was a little more remote than I ordinarily liked to go alone. I had stopped to catch my breath and admire the view of the valley stretched out beneath the mountain. The silence was broken by nearby laughter. Moments later, two women appeared between the scrub along the trail. They were a few years older than me, most likely in their mid-50s, talking, laughing, and having a great time on their morning hike. They stopped to chat for a few minutes. After pointing out that they loved my *fuck cancer* baseball cap, one woman revealed that she was a 4-year survivor of anal cancer; the other a 5-year survivor of breast cancer. They possessed that supernatural ability to connect with another cancer survivor out in the wild.

We spent some time there on the trail exchanging stories about our experiences. But it was what they did not say that made the bigger impression on me. It was clear to see that they were vibrant and healthy. They said they felt more alive now than before they had cancer. I looked forward to the day when I would be all those things again. I knew it was possible because there they stood, perfect examples appearing like apparitions out of the morning fog when I needed them the most.

•   •   •   •   •

When my brother, Todd, and I were in junior high, we convinced our parents that we could go into the Haunted Fun House in Niagara Falls without them. We were old enough and brave enough. We entered the maze like two pre-teen warriors. Once inside the maze, we froze, holding on to each other as if actual mortal dangers awaited us down the darkened corridors. We stood there immobile for so long that a young couple came in. The guy led the way, using the flash on his camera to light up the dark passage at intervals. We could see the scary stuff before we got to it. In the glaring white light of the flashbulb, the so-called scary stuff was ridiculous. Todd and I came through the haunted maze unscathed, with an amusing story to tell.

That was how chemo felt: like a funhouse maze. Since I could not see the twists and turns in the dark, I expected nightmarish phantasms waiting for me around every corner. This time, it was Ella and Alice who provided the flashes of light that revealed my imagined monsters to be far worse than the real ones. I could do this. I may have come through chemo clinging desperately to Louis for courage, but I lived to tell the tale.

Although alone on this journey, people who loved me and genuinely wanted to see me get through this ordeal in one piece surrounded me. They held me up, both physically and emotionally.

During the 10 months of my primary treatments, three friends lost family members to cancer, six friends received new cancer diagnoses, and another moved on to experimental trials when she ran out of treatment options. I struggled with guilt in the face of these realities. It was natural to think, *I'm so thankful that's not me*. I needed the strength to be compassionate when called upon to support others. It was also difficult to resist being dragged down into the sadness and despair of countless others around me in the infusion center who were visibly languishing under the effects of their disease.

Focusing on other people helped me get through this. "There are always people worse off than you." Ordinarily, this is a trite and insensitive thing to say. But it was one of the more important lessons I learned during this experience. I was not looking at other cancer patients with pity or using them to bolster my ego. Their presence reminded me that empathy and decency are of the utmost importance if we are to get through these deadly treatments — and this thing we call life.

The least bit of human connection makes both people feel better, even if that moment is fleeting. The benefit to me was immeasurable. I used every opportunity to reach out and connect with other patients. Maybe we just talked in the elevator, or I held the bathroom door in the infusion ward for someone. It helped me, too. If I was shaking and barely able to stand, I felt that power of connection when other patients reached out to me. Although I was resistant at first, being able to connect with other cancer patients proved to be one of my most important coping mechanisms.

Like weddings, cancer makes shit float to the surface. My perception of the people around me has shifted. I have zero tolerance for insincerity, posers, bullshit, excuses, and laziness. I felt the bitter sting of abandonment from those who I thought were friends but who disappeared at the first sign of trouble. I distanced myself from toxic people and situations. Life is too short for pretense and arrogance.

I became more direct with the people in my life. On the positive side, that meant telling them how much their friendship meant to me, showing gratitude for the slightest gestures, and letting them know how much they are loved. The things that are actually important in my life are not *things* at all. When my life hung in the balance, I was not lying in the hospital bed thinking about money or my career, I only thought about Andrew, Louis, my family, my friends and my dogs. I promised myself I would never make the mistake of worrying about social constructs again. My energies were better spent focused on people and living my fullest life.

Social media cancer comes decorated with trendy wristbands and hashtags: #cancerwarrior #yougotthis #cancersurvivor #fuckcancer. Social media encourages us to craft posts expertly built on manipulative camera filters and gimmicks, but cancer wipes all that fake stuff away instantly. Laying myself bare to my blog readers forced me to take an honest look at myself. I have never regretted this decision. It gave me a second chance to craft a better Lisa in real life. I can never go back to the person I was before.

DREAM EGGS

Louis loves hummingbirds. He hung three hummingbird feeders on our patio. He became obsessed with finding the correct and healthiest food (he even recruited me to make homemade nectar) and was always on a mission to get the perfect photo of their hovering dance.

It is easy to tell which birds are the males, even without getting a close look at the colors of their tiny feathers, because those are the ones that claim a feeder as their own. One little male, who I assume is in charge of our yard, will land on a high branch in our old olive tree to keep watch on all three feeders at once. If any other hummingbird dares to drink from one of *his* feeders, he swoops down mercilessly upon them. I find it fun to watch, but Louis worries the other birds are not getting enough to drink. He put up a fourth feeder just in case.

To me, hummingbirds just sort of appear out of nowhere. For all I knew, hummingbirds are born out of flowers. Other birds make nests we can easily find. A pair of mourning doves used to build their nest, year after year, in the rafters of our covered patio. We witnessed the entire life cycle, from egg to fledgling. We watched a couple of chicks fall to their deaths; I kept another, who survived the fall, in a little box. When it recovered and started flapping its wings again, I placed it near the nest for the parents to find. One year, a Cooper's Hawk killed one, leaving behind a pile of bloody feathers in the backyard. That was a hard lesson for me in observing nature, not intervening, and not getting too upset in the process.

My yoga-slash-music room faces our neighbor's yard. On their side, a wall of dense green trees lines the shared brick fence. With less than 6 feet separation, I see only leaves through my window; my room always has a greenish light about it, like a deep forest.

In the spring, six months before my diagnosis, I was practicing yoga when I noticed a hummingbird showing a lot of interest in a particular branch right outside my window. Multiple times during the hour, I watched her sit on the branch, do something and then fly away. Was it possible that I was witnessing a hummingbird building her nest?

Before this, I had never seen a hummingbird nest in real life. They are impossibly small (about the size of a walnut) and made of spiderwebs. Trying to look at the hummingbird in her nest was like suffering from night blindness. I found it impossible to *see* the bird until I averted my eyes slightly to one side. That was when she revealed herself: a tiny little rust-colored hummingbird sitting on a tiny little nest which would soon hold tiny little eggs. Because I spent a good portion of each day in that room, I got to know this bird intimately. She never moved from that spot. She might be tiny, but her devotion was epic.

I looked forward to seeing her every day. I would stand at the window and look at her before beginning my morning yoga practice. While I was playing my cello each afternoon, I would watch her watching nothing in particular. I liked to think that the positive energy created by my yoga practice and the vibrations of the cello attracted her to my window specifically. She was my friend. She was someone I could count on every day.

It never crossed my mind that the neighbor's gardeners might trim the backs of those trees until the day I arrived home from an errand to see their truck parked out front and to hear the tools running. "No, no, no!!" Running through the house and out the back door, I was in disbelief at what was happening. They had trimmed the entire row of trees. Surely, they had destroyed the hummingbird's nest.

Balancing precariously on my side of the brick wall, I climbed up, getting the gardener's attention. I wanted help with looking around on the ground beneath where I knew the nest to be. "It's going to be about this big," making a circle with my thumb and forefinger. It was hard to hide my panic from them, but I was desperate to find the nest.

After searching for a few minutes, we found the nest, still attached to the severed branch. But it was empty. My heart was in my throat: what had been in the nest? Running some quick calculations, I decided that if there had been any eggs, then the incubation had not yet crossed the two-week mark. I hoped they were still just eggs and not tiny featherless hatchlings who were now trampled under the gardeners' boots.

I knew there was no chance we would find eggs or chicks among the piles of leaves and branches. Even if we had found the eggs, it would have made no difference. The mother was gone, and I was no substitute. It was over. It was still gut-wrenching to decide that it was time to stop looking. I thanked them for taking the time to help me and for at least finding the nest. I climbed back over the wall, the branch and nest in hand. Louis found me in tears on the patio.

How could I explain why I was so upset? He knows me so well. It would be a while before I stopped crying over the tragedy that had just played out. But it was more than just lost eggs. It was the injustice of the death of innocent little birds. And for no good reason. The gardeners were not malicious nor out to kill hummingbird babies that day. We just have this ridiculous need to trim our trees into manicured, unnatural shapes. Their ultimate crime is touching a brick wall. These were unnecessary deaths caused by humans. The dove that the Cooper's hawk had taken would have felt nothing as winged death slammed into her from above. I can reconcile that death. But these hummingbird eggs, so close to hatching, contained tiny birds who would die in the dirt before they were even born.

I thought about this miniature tragedy a lot during my cancer experience. The eggs were the mother hummingbird's dreams canceled. In nature, animals move on with their lives, with more eggs, more kits or cubs, and they put the unexpected tragedies behind them. Multiple attempts every year at reproduction represent the hope of continuing on. Those eggs, that she nurtured and warmed and devoted all her energy to for 14 days, were gone in an instant. All her efforts in this cycle were for nothing. She would not be spending the next month feeding and caring for new babies. Instead, she would have to find her mate again and build a new nest. She was forced, by no fault of her own, to start over from scratch. And unlike most of us humans, she would do it without complaint or self-pity.

Each time it seemed like treatments were going well, my dream eggs were incubating, and I thought I could breathe easily, cancer would come along again to smash them all away. My tiny dream eggs were lost in a pile of cut branches and trampled heartlessly. My heart, the empty nest, left aching for something to wish for.

Like the hummingbird, I had to find a safer spot to build my new nest as I started over again. With every setback there grew within me, the determination to be stronger. I learned to walk away from the things that can never be and to be fearless as I rebuild.

Cancer has made me more realistic, while revealing the world to be more mysterious. I stopped questioning *why* and accepted that some things just *are*. What a relief to know that I do not need to have all the answers and explanations. I took my medicine, and the tumor died. It is enough to celebrate that the drugs worked; no need to understand all the science behind them.

With each new set of tiny dream eggs, I learned patience and perseverance. When I look through the lens of alacrity at my life with cancer, I have had more dream eggs turn into little birds than have not. There is a lot to celebrate.

·　　·　　·　　·　　·

Fighting cancer was the loneliest thing I have ever done. Even among the dozens of people in the infusion center, it was still a solo flight. Family and friends with the best intentions try to connect with us, but cancer patients are ultimately alone. The specter of death haunts each of us, binding us together like huddling rabbits. We are the few people who understand what it means to be alone together. Bonding with other cancer patients and survivors is so important for getting through this. With their support, friendship, and love, I found the strength to put one shaky foot in front of the other and sometimes even offer that same support to others who needed it.

No one wants to be a member of Cancer Club. One day, we find ourselves being forced into it. We move among everyone else unnoticed, though there is an instant recognition when we cross paths out in the wild. Friends and family who are cancer survivors immediately attach to us, supporting us in ways we never imagined possible.

I often wondered if Cancer Club members could still recognize one another after treatments were over, when we were no longer wearing the uniform. I got my answer to this question a few weeks after chemotherapy, when I could drive myself to one of my appointments at the cancer center. A woman held the elevator for me. "You don't need to hurry. I've got the door for you!" I thanked her and stepped into the elevator to stand next to her. She started making small talk and judging by what she was saying, she was a cancer survivor herself. She may have had an easier time identifying me because of my bald head, but I recognized a fellow traveler, too. It was nice to see someone thriving. In just one 60-second elevator ride, she infused me with multiple weeks of inspiration.

Every two weeks, as I walked through the ward to my favorite corner cubicle to receive my treatments, I passed by the other patients receiving their medicines. Some had the curtain drawn; others left it open so they could watch the activity of the nurses and volunteers. I always found this interesting. I wanted my curtain open, but because of COVID, I always felt safer leaving it shut — one more paper-thin barrier between the virus and my decimated immune system. When my curtain was open, I found the other patients mesmerizing. Sometimes they would return the glance, lock eyes for a moment, and the tops of our faces would soften over our masks. We were not merely smiling at each other. We were communicating: *I know you.*

Often the youngest person in the infusion center, I always felt the eyes of the older patients on me. They never transmitted sympathy. It felt more like antipathy toward cancer itself. The average age of certain cancers is lowering, and I felt their unadulterated frustration at this statistic. Face to face with a younger patient, the injustice of it all hitting home. I understood because this is how I feel about children with cancer.

Even with all the support systems in the world at our disposal: loving partners, doting parents, and compassionate friends, we are still alone in this. No one understands what we are going through, except other people who have been through it.

I was not interested in making friends with any other cancer patients; I was uncharacteristically closed off and private. Another woman in my neighborhood was diagnosed with colon cancer around the same time as me. I dreaded bumping into her on the sidewalk; I wanted to hide from her. There would be no commiserations or get-togethers. I did not want to carry someone else's fears and worries along with my own. My struggle was enough of a burden for me. I did not want to share my cancer with anyone.

I did not want to make any new friends who might not be around for much longer. That frightened me above all. Perhaps I was being selfish, but I was spending so much energy on my survival, I had none to spare on heartbreak.

Talking to other people who had survived their cancers gave me an important perspective from *The Other Side.* They each had faced unique cancers and survived. They were my cheerleaders, and they gave me the tough details that they never told me before I had cancer myself.

I found I did this, as well. I kept the finer details of my diagnosis and my treatments private. When someone asked how I was, I answered with pre-digested answers. "I'm dealing with side effects from chemo," or "My next surgery will be soon," or "It's been rough, but I'm doing better now." But when Ella wanted to know how I was, I could give her the actual answer. "I'm so fucking tired of this…" She knew precisely what *this* was. *This* is something so unspeakably awful that there is no name for it. No one, except other cancer survivors, understands *this*. We need each other. Together, we can cry and rage and moan and celebrate without words.

For many weeks, I mostly avoided making any new cancer friends. By writing the blog I was allowing people into my experience, so I felt relieved of the duty to join in on someone else's. I wanted to be left alone in my misery. I was hoarding my cancer like Gollum and *The Ring* and isolating myself much the same way.

When I met Suzy at the infusion center, I was terrified to the point of feeling sick; terrified to get attached to someone; terrified to open myself up to someone; terrified to have to touch and feel and be with another real cancer patient. It was our nurses, Abby and Terry, who decided that we needed each other as part of our care plans.

Terry was the one to fetch me from my cubicle before Suzy and I began our infusions that morning. Despite my best efforts up to this point, I fell head over heels for Suzy. All my tough talk about not wanting to meet other cancer patients flew out the window. Here I was, allowing a deep attachment to take hold with that first conversation.

Suzy was 44 and had Stage-4 Colon Cancer. Though I often felt like her cancer was much more insidious than mine. She had no intestinal symptoms when she saw her doctor about a mysterious lump in her neck. This turned out to be a metastasis from a mystery cancer. Only after a battery of scans and tests did they discover she had colon cancer. She did not have surgery before chemo, and unlike me, she made the heartbreaking decision to ask Dr. Jacobs what her prognosis was. With a 6-year-old son to tether her to life, she had to live with an exponentially larger amount of fear and uncertainty in her already heavily burdened soul.

My Cancer Train had stopped at this station and Suzy was getting on board. We were now alone together in this messed up train car. But I am so thankful, every single day since that morning, that cancer brought together us.

We talked for longer than we realized — both our nurses were hovering at a polite distance as a gentle reminder we needed to get started with our infusions. It was with much reluctance that we hugged and wished each other good luck for the day. I returned to my corner room.

I never wanted to feel sorry for anyone with cancer, and I did not want anyone feeling sorry for me. Sending negative energy like that does no one any good. Instead, I tried to flip it around and feel empathy and send as much healing strength as I could spare. I did not feel sorry for Suzy. The unfairness of her having cancer enraged me. I wanted Suzy to have the strength to beat this thing. She was always on my mind, regardless of how awful I was feeling during my infusion. I would ask the nurses for reports. "Is Suzy doing ok?" Every time my curtain opened, I would try to get a glance toward her cubicle to see if hers was open, too.

This infusion was the most difficult one for me. Lightheaded and drowsy, I spent most of the morning with my eyes closed, head in my hands. Louis had his hands full with me during a tough trip to the bathroom — I was dizzy and weak and nearly fell trying to get up off the toilet. We came out to find Suzy leaning against the wall. She looked barely conscious. I could hardly stand up myself. Walking was so difficult during this infusion that I clung to Louis and the IV tree like a toddler between parents. But I was more concerned about Suzy and if she was ok there alone, her IV tree her only support. I reached out, and she reached back, finding each other in the dark funhouse. Silently, we held hands there in the hallway, transparent shells of the people we had been just a couple of hours earlier. Alone together, bonded and floating in this sea of misery, no words were necessary to convey the horrors going on inside of us.

I thought of her for the next 46 hours while I was home with my pump. Doing this gave me the strength to make it through that infusion. Two days later, when I returned to have my 5-FU pump removed, I did not have the chance to see Suzy again, as I was there a couple of hours ahead of her. But I wanted her to know I was thinking of her. I made her a gift bag, inspired by all the empowering gifts I had received from friends, which I left with the nurses to give to her when she returned later that day to have her pump removed. Suzy would probably not reach out, but I put my phone number and email address in a card, anyway. It did not matter to me if she kept in touch, just as long as she knew that channel was open if she needed to talk.

She reached out, and we texted each other virtually every day. I saw Suzy several times over the next few weeks, sometimes before our infusions, and sometimes before our office visits. We never said hello, we only threw ourselves into each other's arms like two survivors of a shipwreck, holding on with all the waning strength we could muster, desperate to not face this horror alone.

After finishing her first 12 weeks of chemo and getting the results of her PET scan, the doctors decided she would need another six doses of the drugs. She faced her second 12 weeks of chemotherapy with stoic grace and determination. Although my heart broke for her, I refused to inject any sort of panic or negativity into her already difficult situation. I sat with her during several of her infusions over the following months, while I was going through radiation. We spent countless hours crying, hugging, raging, holding hands, and laughing together, enjoying these reunions, and always feeling like there was never enough time.

More than once, we apologized to the nurses for making so much noise in the quiet infusion center. Terry responded, "Don't stop! Hearing your laughter is like music."

All of us mothers with cancer share the same unspeakable fears regarding leaving our children behind. This is a fear so awful I never want to talk about it. Despite my own deep anxieties, just knowing that Suzy carried these same worries in her soul, fearing that she may not live long enough to see her son start high school, devastated me. I have never experienced such a strong desire for someone else to be well. I want Suzy to beat this thing and to watch her son grow up. I want her to find peace and joy and love in this precious life we temporarily enjoy.

With all my heart, I want Suzy, and every single one of her dream eggs, to live.

PART THREE

Fate shouted to the warrior, "You cannot withstand the storm!"
The warrior whispered back, "I am the storm."
– Unknown

PATIENT 28448

According to a wave of articles in 2022, all cancers, including colorectal cancer, are on the rise among younger and middle-aged adults[14]. During this year, I watched as cancer also affected multiple friends. Too many of them in their 40s and 50s diagnosed with various forms of the disease. For those of us in the *Sandwich Generation,* cancer comes at a most inopportune period of our lives. We have college-age children gaining independence and aging parents who are losing theirs; in the prime of our careers, we balance the responsibilities of owning a home and being productive members of society. The pause in our middle years causes many issues that can reverberate throughout the remaining decades of our lives.

For younger adults, another set of stressful issues comes into play. Many reports show that cancer patients in their 20s are likely to lack proper health insurance coverage if they have any at all. There is a low likelihood that they have hundreds of thousands of dollars in savings to pay for treatments not covered by their inadequate insurance. This could force them

---

[14] https://www.cancer.org/latest-news/study-finds-sharp-rise-in-colon-cancer-and-rectal-cancer-rates-among-young-adults.html

to work through a very serious illness like cancer, causing their financial futures to be saddled with debt from medical bills, which are already buried under crushing student loans. The intense stress of finding financial stability after recovery could contribute to the recurrence of cancer. It can also increase the risk of a new cancer later in life.

I have read several health institution sources — including medical journals, which I had to use Google to translate back into English — that talk about the *whole patient* and the potential for suffering years beyond remission from the effects of having cancer at the start of life. This is serious business. How can we fix this? How can we help those younger people for the rest of their long lives?

At my age, there was an ever-present stress surrounding my career simmering under the surface. I know I had more important things to focus on, like living. But it was impossible to shelve the worry that I might not be able to get back to work after this. Many cancer patients can apply for government help like unemployment and disability programs, take medical leaves of absence from their workplace, and sometimes continue to work from home while enduring their treatments. The music business is unlike most other career paths. There are no work-from-home orchestras. A freelance musician, I was wholly unemployed for over a year with no recourse.

Because freelance work involves word-of-mouth hiring and recommendations, I risked being forgotten. This was a legitimate fear surrounding my work. Would I have a career to return to when this was over? Would I have to start from square one or might some generous contacts hire me as if no time had passed? I only hoped to practice my cello, even through the painful Hand and Foot Syndrome, so that when I broke out of cancer jail, I would be ready to work.

As children, our parents and teachers tell us that being *unique* is such an important thing to be. Which is great when that applies to artistic talent or math abilities, fashion style and haircuts, personalities, and gymnastic skills. I am relieved that I was not a unique cancer case. Being a vanilla, boring, textbook medical case is always the way to go. *Basic run-of-the-mill colon cancer* was a known entity to all the medical professionals involved in my treatment. It would have been a different story if just one doctor had reacted shocked or stumped or worried.

I have learned a lot about how the medical system works through stories from friends and family. Talk to anyone who has had cancer, and they will confirm that their journey was not just a simple path of diagnosis-treatment-remission-the-end. It is a complicated, many-layered, and private situation which very few people can appreciate from the outside looking in. After my diagnosis, it shocked me to learn how many of my friends and colleagues had survived cancer, because most of them went through the journey in private.

Until I went through it myself, I was unaware of the sprawling landscape of cancer treatments and procedures. I always thought people had chemo or radiation, and that was it. So, when I was first navigating the waters, I was woefully uneducated and completely overwhelmed by all the information coming at me. Friends who I had not known were cancer survivors selflessly reached out to lend emotional support. They translated the medical mumbo-jumbo in a way that I could understand without being frightened out of my mind. The weeks pressed on, and they opened up about their own experiences. I always felt like their information revealed itself in onion layers, telling me the awful details only when I hit certain milestones. They would text me when I needed support, a form of ESP that binds us together on a different plane. This ability to bond with other cancer survivors is what can save our sanity, and more importantly, our lives.

When people feel safe enough to open up, they make themselves accessible. Not like when I was a child. Back then, people would whisper the word *cancer*. They tried to keep us kids in the dark, protecting us from the scary reality. But there is still a tendency to avoid talking about it with someone who has it. When someone has had cancer or has seen a loved one go through it, then all bets are off.

My fear surrounding my increasing pain and an uncertain diagnosis was growing in the fall of 2021, and I found myself drawn to Ella like a moth to a flame. Something inside me told me she would be an important emotional force, and I needed to let her in. And when I did, she took on a role much like a big sister. She soothed my fears yet remained lucid about what was happening to me. Although she is very protective of her private life, she laid herself bare to me about her cancer experience and our friendship deepened thanks to this horrible disease.

Ella was a pillar of strength for me in those weeks before my diagnosis, when I was at my most fearful. She would remind me that there was no use in freaking out. Just hold on to the *facts* of what the doctors were telling me. Do not let my imagination get the better of me. I am certain that she knew I was going to be diagnosed with cancer long before I even contemplated the possibility.

She continuously reminded me that everything happening to me was out of my control. "The only thing that's certain with cancer is that things will change quickly and unexpectedly."

This advice was invaluable to me after the surgery following chemo when Dr. Quilici discovered the remaining cancerous implants in my pelvis. In fact, her advice proved true throughout the whole of my experience.

The human element of medical care is as important as the scientific side. After my diagnosis, I signed into my new hospital portal, where I could view all my test results and confirm upcoming appointments. Pretty straightforward and dry stuff. There was an option to add a personal profile picture. Knowing every doctor and nurse who signed in to access my records would see it, I settled on a photo, taken a few months before my diagnosis. *Crow Pose.* A strong and dynamic arm balance, I thought it looked impressive in the tiny circle of space allotted for the profile picture. No way could I have predicted just how significant this photo choice was going to be. Every single person who accessed my files at the hospital and cancer center always commented on how amazing that photo was. Over the course of the next year, I would change that photo on a monthly basis to more current ones that showed off my bald head, colostomy bag, and thinning body. But always featuring an impressive yoga pose.

Our doctors and nurses see us at our worst, often in a baggy hospital gown, and altogether unrecognizable. I wanted them all to see *me.* They needed to know *who* they were treating and to feel something about me. Using those pictures was probably one of the better instincts I had.

The Team of Grownups (Dr. Kagan, Dr. Quilici, and Dr. Jacobs) always made me feel like they saw me. I was not a nameless patient sitting on the exam table with a just file number to identify me; they knew who I was as a whole person. I always felt they were intent on saving the person, not just curing the body. We all have a rich life worth saving. Specialists, who might only meet with me once, could find it difficult to get to know me. So, it was important that I had a deeper relationship with my primary physician. Dr. Kagan was a powerful advocate when I needed a voice. He set me up with specialists he believed would be the most receptive to me and my situation in a short amount of time. His referrals to Dr. Quilici and Dr. Jacobs were like the most successful blind dates in history.

By contrast, I felt like Dr. Messina and Dr. Unger only viewed me as a two-dimensional case file, and they were only looking at the symptoms that concerned them and their specialty: female age 47 presents with pain to lower left pelvic quadrant *blah blah blah* history of endometriosis peri menopausal *yadda yadda yadda* laxative recommended to relieve constipation. Cured! Send in the next patient.

They never asked the most basic, getting to know you, questions: what I did for a living, how long Louis and I had been married, how many kids we had. They did not even know in which part of Los Angeles we lived. Not even a single question about my tattoos. Every doctor and nurse on my new team asks about the beautiful king snake tattoo on my right forearm. Brian, a nurse in Dr. Jacobs' office, loves to compare our tattoos while he draws my blood. To me, it just seems like an obvious conversation starter; an easy way to get to know someone. I am not a biker chick; I am a classical musician with lots of tattoos that I love to talk about. Done. Patient #28448 now has a unique trait that sets her apart from the parade of other patients that day.

When a man in his 60s walks into the doctor's office complaining of chest pain, they send him straight to the ER under the assumption he is having a heart attack. If a 77-year-old woman has severe back pain, the doctor assumes she may have fractured her back. A decade ago, a 38-year-old colleague of mine complained of a chronic cough to his doctor; he was told he just had a bad chest cold. He declined rapidly, progressing from bronchitis to pneumonia to dead within just a couple of weeks because pneumonia was not on the doctor's radar. What if he had been 83? Would pneumonia have been at the top of the list?

This is like my experience with the doctor two decades ago who blew off my rectal bleeding as hemorrhoids. If someone had known it was extensive endometriosis sooner, they would have spared me many years of pain, suffering, and anxiety. I should have been more closely examined or sent to a specialist sooner. I was too young to know of the existence of medical-advocacy and the importance of second opinions. Endometriosis is not a life-threatening condition. But what if it had been something more serious? I was in my early 20s, but that did not mean that I was immune from life-threatening diseases.

Thankfully, when I went to Dr. Kagan complaining of pain, we had enough of a relationship for him to know what behaviors were normal for me. I am not one to blow pain out of proportion. I am not a hypochondriac. I only visited the office for my yearly physical or when something was actually wrong with me. I am a very healthy and very energetic person. When I showed up looking like a wet dog with sad drooping ears and heavy eyelids, he knew something was wrong. A specialist like Dr. Quilici never met me before I was that sad dog. He did not see the *real me* until months after he had already performed several surgeries on me. He never knew me as I actually am. Yet he always treated me as if I were a healthy person. Now that he has gotten to know me better over the many months of my treatment, he has a clearer picture of who I am. This has already proven useful in his assessments of my surgical recoveries. Dr. Jacobs met me at my lowest as well, and week after week saw my cycles of chemo and recovery until eventually, he saw actual recovery. He questioned me, week after week, for nearly a year,

"Are you able to practice your yoga?" Certainly, choosing a profile picture that portrayed me at my best, helped.

Throughout my treatment, I always got the impression that the doctors took a personal interest in me. I chalked this up to excellent bedside manner. Louis theorized they were fond of me. One nurse offered, "You must have good karma." Whatever the reason, it came as no surprise that Dr. Jacobs would hold my chemo-burnt and peeling hands in his while he spoke to me, petting them in the most caring way; that Dr. Quilici would squeeze my shoulder at the end of each visit; or that when my diagnosis seemed imminent, and I was at my most terrified, Dr. Kagan hugged me and said, "Don't worry. We're all going to take good care of you."

This is what Human Medicine looks like.

THE BELL

I awoke on Friday, March 18, 2022, filled with excitement. The last day of my chemotherapy had finally arrived. The only thing left to do was to get the pump removed and ring the bell. Chemotherapy would officially be over. Months earlier, Dr. Jacobs had stood at my hospital bedside and told me the regimen would be 12 weeks. He may as well have said 12 years. Looking ahead at chemo is a lot different from looking back on it. It had passed in the blink of an eye.

Everyone who completes chemotherapy knows about *The Bell*. During the previous three months, I clapped and cheered for other patients as they rang the bell, so my anticipation and excitement to do the same had been growing.

"Today I get to ring the bell!" Riding the morning surge of energy, I showered and got ready for the appointment. I felt like a little kid excited about a trip to Disneyland. I had not been sleeping much for the last four weeks. Acid reflux, a side effect of the drugs, made it difficult to lie down. And yet on this morning, I was full of energy for no good reason.

It was after that initial thrill that a familiar dark cloud came over me. After my shower, seeing my naked body in the mirror revealed the true extent of cancer's effect on me — the pump over my shoulder, the colostomy bag stuck to my abdomen, and all the tracks of scars in my pasty white skin. For the first time, I allowed myself to take a thorough look in the mirror and not shy away from what cancer and chemotherapy had done to my body. I needed to take a photo of this moment.

I was constantly reminding myself that *chemo is saving my life*, and *this is all temporary*. But, when I stopped to see the changes in my body, all I felt was resentment toward the drugs. I had been doing pretty darn good before this stupid cancer thing. It felt like my old reflection would never return.

I hated the image, but this was the exact sort of photo I needed to post on my blog. Despite what I had been posting, chemotherapy had not always been kind to me. It was not business as usual around here. They needed to see that I was thin, pale, bald, and drained. I stood there for all the world to see in a bralette and yoga pants, no scarf over my head to distract from my swollen face, a clear colostomy bag so everyone could see my stoma and some poop, an IV line attached to the portacath in my chest, and every angry red incision visible along with every single rib. This was the most important picture I took of myself during my cancer treatments.

This was what having cancer looked like.

Chemo was gnarly as fuck. It was important for people to see the truth of it all. I have never, in my life, had to hold my shit together like this and for such a long period. I could go a few days, convinced that I was doing well. But then out of the blue, rage, fear, and sadness would overtake me, and I would collapse into a heap. The next moment, I would pull myself together and act as if nothing had happened.

This experience with chemo was unique to me. Several colon cancer survivors in my support group told me they could not tolerate all 6 doses of FOLFIRINOX and had to be taken off the drugs; Alice suffered a severe reaction during her first infusion and was given an oral chemotherapy drug instead. Suzy had fewer side effects than I did. But the ones she had were more intense. Although her cancer and chemotherapy differed from mine, Ella's ability to tolerate her drugs waned and during her final infusion, she had to be rushed to the ICU. I wondered which was worse: having a laundry list of side effects at a tolerable level like I did, or only a few at a deadly level.

I went into this whole crazy ride with my eyes *wide open*. I only expected I would be forced to dig deep for the strength and courage to get through the treatments, which I did one day, one hour, or sometimes one never-ending minute at a time. No one knows how their chemotherapy will affect their body until they are in it. I certainly did not. I scared myself silly imagining my first infusion. Although I experienced everything in glaring technicolor, the memories are painted in fuzzy, grey, broad strokes. The smaller details of the side effects lost in time. They faded, just like the memory of labor pains after having a baby. Thankfully, I had written all my side effects in my journal while I was experiencing them because there are many I have no recollection of now. It still shocks me to read it, but then I think, *yeah, I guess it really was that rough.* No wonder I lost my mind now and again.

Dr. Jacobs wrote me a prescription for the anti-anxiety medication Ativan, but I never took a single pill. Instead, I relied heavily on marijuana. Feeling nauseous? Zofran did its job well, but a puff of marijuana hurried along the effects of the drug while putting me in a more reasonable state of mind. After a little pot, I could feel the anxiety melting away. I could calm down after a hysterical cry and take a step back from the situation to reassure myself *it's ok, you're ok, just breathe.*

Cancer burns raw, delicate, open wounds in our souls. It has meant so much to me when Alice or Ella soothed me. They knew what I was going through, because they had been through the same thing. "You'll get through this even though it doesn't feel possible right now." We do not *need* permission to flip out, but sometimes it helps to have it. More than once, Ella listened quietly as I cried over the phone. It is unthinkable that either of them would ever utter the words, "Don't worry, it'll be ok," because it is inconceivable. They know better than anyone else: nothing will *ever* be ok.

People want to fix every single emotion someone they love is having. Whether they are uncomfortable watching us cry, or the emotion of fear is too intense for them to handle, no one likes to see someone else in turmoil. Their first reaction is to want to cure us of it. What they never consider is that we might not want to be fixed.

With cancer, it is essential to sob until we are gasping for breath, hiccupping and gagging; to cry until we are so exhausted that we pass out; to yell and pound or kick something; to stand in the shower and weep for no reason; to pull a blanket over our head, curl up into a ball, and moan into the pillow. A loving partner gets under the blanket and, without saying a word, lays there with us until it passes.

My emotional state looked more like an abstract splatter of paints vandalizing a classic Degas, imposing an indecipherable hot mess of incompetence over a priceless scene of graceful ballerinas. There is no fixing the inner turmoil of a cancer patient. And that *is* ok.

My biggest regret is not pushing harder for Louis to find more support to help him through this whole thing. He is an intensely private person. Although there were people who offered to be there for him, I knew he would never accept that kind of attention. I only had a peripheral knowledge of what he was doing to get the emotional support that he needed, which mostly involved talking to a close friend and working on that bottle of Ativan that I was ignoring. I had limited energy to devote to making sure everyone around me was doing ok. I had to trust that this was enough for him.

Finishing with chemotherapy must have come as a tremendous relief to Louis. As I rang the bell, celebrating my survival, he must have felt he had broken through the surface of a fathomless ocean. He could breathe the fresh air again.

THE SHIRT

Three weeks after I finished chemotherapy, I stood in my closet looking for something to wear like I do every single morning. I came across the shirt I wore during each one of my infusions. My chemo-uniform. I started to shake, my palms got sweaty, and my throat closed as waves of nausea crashed over me. *What was going on? Was it possible to react so strongly to a piece of clothing?*

Overcome with revulsion, I ripped the shirt off the hanger and threw it on the floor. There was no plan for what I was going to do with it. I only knew that I wanted it to suffer. I looked down at it like a piece of garbage polluting my closet. After stomping on it a few times, I kicked the shirt out the door and into the bathroom. I stared at it with contempt while I got dressed, wondering what punishment it deserved next.

I texted Lori, "Is it weird that the chemo shirt makes me feel like puking?"

Without skipping a beat, she texted me back, "No, throw it out."

I wanted this thing out of my life. After kicking the shirt around the bathroom floor a couple more times for good measure, I clawed at it with my hands. I pulled and stretched it as far as my arms could reach. My veins flooded with satisfaction as the seams popped and ripped. If I could have, I would have torn it up with my teeth. Just like Dusty had chewed and destroyed the cone, getting rid of this shirt was my catharsis.

Because fuck that shirt, and fuck cancer.

SPRING

One of the weirder things I had to adjust to when I moved to Southern California is that the Canada Geese migrate backward. I spent the first 32 years of my life in New England, where geese flying south in V formations overhead in September signaled the coming winter. Their departure always brought on a sort of melancholy. Although they spent their summers chasing me on my bike, nipping at my feet, while the toddler Andrew squealed with equal parts delight and terror from the baby seat, I was sorry to see them leave. The cold months were coming, and our feathered friends were abandoning us.

Winters are much quieter in the northeast. Only a few bird species hang in there, braving the elements. Those that stay keep rather silent. Nestled at the bottom of Pine Cobble in the Berkshire Mountains, my storybook 1850s' Victorian looked out on a picturesque New England view. Our property sloped up toward the mountain, which meant we could take Andrew sledding in our own backyard. A creek wound its way through the patchwork of lush green trees that covered the gentle slope of the mountain. In the winter, the creek froze over, and the trees were grey skeletal sentinels covered in snow.

Cardinals were some of the only winter birds remaining. When one landed on an icy tree branch, it was like a bloodstain on white lace. My eyes could see nothing else except that point of color, and it was difficult to tear my attention away. A sign of life in a hibernating world. Are there cardinals here in Los Angeles? If there are, I have yet to see any. I miss them.

The honking geese return to Southern California in October, their arrival instead signaling the start of winter. I often joke that there is not a real winter here. Louis has told me that Los Angeles natives call the season *Not Summer*. It never gets all that cold here. There is not a single real coat in my closet anymore, just a lot of knit cardigans, light fleece vests, and an extensive collection of colorful scarves. Winter here has a yellow-muted sunlight about it, which although it does not drag me down into wistful nostalgia for winters in New England, it still gives me a twinge of calm and sentimentality. It encourages me to slow down a bit, though I do not go into full hibernation mode here as I did back east.

When the vacationing geese run their first practice drills in small battalions for their return migration, usually around the first weeks of March, I get that same old melancholy as they prepare to leave us. Once the flocks decide it is time to go and the giant V's soar overhead in a cacophony of instinct, I get a little sad again. It seems I never want them to leave, no matter where I live, and no matter how aggressive they are on the ground. I like to believe the same geese flying over me here will end up flying over my family and friends thousands of miles away.

It might seem silly, as they go overhead, for me to say, "Good luck! Have a safe trip!" and "See you next year!" But I do it.

When a large group of them flies overhead, I wonder how many will ultimately make it to their destination. Do they mourn the loss of comrades along the way? Naïve as it sounds, I believe wholeheartedly that geese notice when someone leaves their ranks forever. They probably notice it more than we notice the loss.

I like to believe we leave a mark on everyone we encounter. So, it would stand to reason that we should strive toward making those memories positive. A few teachers in my childhood said something so outrageous or did something so shocking that it burned my developing brain; and 40 years later, when I think about it, I get just as outraged as I did when it happened. I remember those teachers just as I remember the exceptional teachers. True to form, those exceptional teachers remain a part of my life. They have been integral to my mental health to survive this cancer thing. The teacher who taught me how to write in complete sentences when I was 7 years old, and the one who taught me how to recognize chords by ear, are cheering me on 40 years later. Only now they are my friends.

I want to be like them. Those teachers have inspired me, when dealing with my music students, to always try to put my best intentions forward. A student may show up for a lesson without practicing their scales, yet, through my frustration, I can still find a compliment for the notes they played correctly. All our students, in fact, everyone we deal with, deserve praise for something. No matter how insignificant I may have thought it was, one kind word could make all the difference to their success as adults. When I send positivity out into the world, I receive it back exponentially. Many of my former students have kept in touch with me over the years, sending me photos of their own children.

I have never thrown away any gifts my students have given me over these (almost) 30 years of my career. In my yoga-slash-music room, I have an impressive collection of figurines, jewelry, high school graduation and wedding photos, and scraps of paper with smiley faces drawn on them. My Christmas tree boasts several ornaments, and my kitchen cabinets are full of coffee mugs. I never erase the marks they have made in the music they borrowed from me. I have a book of duets in which several bear the tag: "Sam's Favorite" in swirly girly handwriting. Years later, opening a page to play one of those duets with a new student, I am flush with a wave of joy when they ask, "Who's Sam?" Being able to share the story of one of my very first students from almost thirty years ago with a new one makes me feel like she is still with me somehow.

I cherish the memories of her, and all the kids I have taught over the years. I just wish I could remember Samantha's last name.

Going through cancer, sometimes people acted as if I were already dead — afraid to use the word *cancer* or worse, they avoided talking to me about the future. This is a big deal, actually. Many cancer patients might be afraid to think about the future, so they avoid making plans. They never allow themselves to count on anything or anyone. But there are fleeting moments when we unconsciously talk about *next month* or *next year*. These are all signs that we sense healing is happening and life will go on.

I was never afraid to plan. I never reached a point where I was reluctant to talk about *the summer* or *next year*. It was always just a matter-of-fact thing for me. In February, only three infusions into my treatment, I was making plans for the spring months immediately following the last treatment in March. I even signed up for a 5K race in June. I never avoided thinking about the future. My participation in life months down the line was never in question. Even if I had to cancel or change my plans, I had no hesitation in making them in the first place.

My future is no more uncertain than any other person on this planet. A perfectly healthy person could get hit by a car tomorrow and a child with supposedly incurable cancer could live to be 90. Life automatically comes with a terminal diagnosis. We know nothing of our fate.

The geese arrived here in Southern California just as I was about to get my diagnosis, and they were packing up to leave six months later as chemo was ending. Seemed appropriate. Winter was hard, but spring was coming, and life would return to normal. This year, as they flew overhead, it reminded me that life continues regardless of what was going on in my tiny insignificant human life. I found deep comfort in knowing that nothing outside of my tiny world had changed.

Kiki is one of my dearest friends here in Los Angeles. One of the first people I met when I moved here in 2010, we were instant friends. For most of the intervening years, we got together every week to practice yoga. We continued to do this through both her pregnancies, and then practiced over Zoom video calls during the COVID lockdown. In nearly 10 years, we did not miss a single week until I started having chronic pain and was canceling on her more often than not. Even when I showed up to practice, my first complaint was about how much pain I was having. She was correctly concerned and lent me immeasurable support during that scary time.

I missed her with every fiber of my being during treatment, even though she stopped by my house every week. She had to stay in her car while I stood in my driveway, handing me loaves of warm, homemade rustic bread through her car window. I was thankful for the opportunity to say hello to her. But that was about as close as we could get to one another for over four months.

She texted me one morning in April, as I neared the six-week post-chemo mark, to ask if she could come over to drop off another loaf of bread. I told her I could do her one better: we can meet on my patio for a proper visit.

When she came around the corner of the house, I burst into tears. My ankles hurt, my legs were wobbly, and I had a limp that made it look like I was perpetually walking downhill. I was thinner and older than she remembered. She stepped up on to the patio and I threw myself at her. I just kept repeating into her ear, "I've missed you so much." I was starved for female contact. Women are softer and warmer. We all seem to be natural empaths with each other. We ended up talking and watching her son play in my yard for almost two hours (it is amazing how much a 5-year-old grows in six months) before she had to leave. Of course, I cried again when we said goodbye. I did not realize how much I loved her until I felt my heart ache while we were apart. Seeing her made me appreciate just how much I had missed out on. She, and everyone else, living in a parallel world that had continued without me all those months.

Kiki's arrival at my house was like the cardinal in winter signaling the coming spring. Real life was just around the corner; I would be around my friends, family, and colleagues soon enough. I remembered what Dr. Jacobs had said to me at my darkest moment, "This is all temporary." Three months of chemotherapy did not seem temporary when I was crouched on the starting blocks. It is astounding how quickly time flew by. In the grand arc of my life, those three months of chemotherapy were as insignificant as one winter in a lifetime.

Like perennial seeds sprouting in the garden in spring, signs that my body was recovering were emerging. At eight weeks post-chemo, my hair filled in the bald spots and my eyelashes were growing back. For the first time in months, I could look in the mirror and see the obvious improvements for myself.

I had shaved my head for what I hoped would be the last time, telling myself that I wanted to keep everything the same length until real growth began. I like neat rows, color-coordinated spreadsheets, written-out lists, Scandinavian furniture, and for all my hair to be the same length.

It took three months before the chemo lines across my thumbnails grew out. Although the cold sensitivity in my hands had lessened, it was still present. Dr. Jacobs expected this to last up to a year. I thought I was being a wuss; I just assumed that after 12 weeks of avoiding touching anything cool, I had PCSD — post chemo stress disorder. Turns out the neuropathy was as real as the lines on my nails.

After the treatment ended, I put back 8 pounds of the weight I had lost. A good sign that the cancer was not sucking calories from me anymore. I knew someday I would miss the days of eating with impunity as I did during cancer treatments, so I tried to enjoy food as much as I could. My tastebuds were growing back, so I was enjoying a more interesting menu again. This would give me a buffer going into surgery and whatever treatment came next.

Obviously, I loved and appreciated Louis' constant vigilant attention and effort to help me through this period of my life, but I was delighted to see him working again in his studio composing and not worrying if it was ok to leave me alone in a different room. He met up with his sons for lunch on the weekends and went hiking without rushing back to check on me. Sometimes he even let me drive alone to my weekly check-ups. All signs that I was being trusted to take care of myself again. This felt great.

I will never moan about doing the laundry, sweeping the patio, cleaning the countertops, or any mundane household chore again. Cancer patients might be the only people in the world who mutter the words "I can't wait to get back to work," with any sincerity. Now that I know what it feels like to be unable to do basic things, I appreciated these as the first signs of spring.

During the cold, dark winter months, my head was bald like the trees. Icy winds blew through the bare branches like the icy drugs coursing through my veins. The season was changing. The springtime sun rising higher in the sky, I was unfurling and reaching for it like a sprouting seed through the thawing soil. Winter was over. I was coming back to life.

RETURNING

The memory of chemotherapy was very peculiar, a stranger's experience. It played in my mind like misaligned View-Master reels, the revolving dioramas snapping into view as double images, and in no particular order. I would think, *I can't believe any of this happened to me*, convinced that I had watched someone else go through the experience. Sometimes my memories of the treatments behaved like almost-forgotten dreams, wisps of fine misty clouds that drifted just outside my periphery. If I tried to look straight at them, they disappeared like the hummingbird in her nest, and leaving me desperate to remember what it looked like.

Maybe someday I will grasp the deeper meaning of this experience. At 47, the mid-point of my life, I wonder if this happened for a reason. What will Lisa from 48 to 100 be like? With her death sentence commuted, what difference will she make in the world? Although lacking a crystal ball, I was pretty sure that once the drugs wore off and the whole cancer thing was growing smaller in the horizon behind me, I would be the same snarky, persnickety, opinionated, insolent person I had always been.

To celebrate the culmination of something as outrageous and inconceivable as chemotherapy, all we do is ring a bell on the last day. They don't hand us *I completed six rounds of chemo and all I got was this lousy T-shirt,* T-shirts and a goody bag. I walked away with the heaviest baggage imaginable which I have to lug with me on every subsequent trip around the sun.

It was impossible to get a handle on the passage of time while I was busy working hard to survive cancer. I measured time by when I met my monthly, weekly, daily, and hourly milestones, and only knew what day of the week it was thanks to my pill dispenser. The world continued without me, perhaps my first actual glimpse of what will happen when I someday die. Life went on without me. I am not as important as I thought I was. It was a relief to be shown I did not need to make myself sick trying to do or be everything.

In the weeks post-chemo, I ran the gamut of emotions from elation to despair, from joy to mourning, and from optimism to outright terror. It would be impossible for anyone to go through this experience without being affected at every turn. Getting a bit of good news can bring about intense tears while bad news rendered me emotionless. I could no longer predict what reaction I would have to anything anymore.

My post-chemo recovery period came with a new set of emotions. The relief of finishing treatment passed right away, replaced with the anxiety of the *what-ifs* flooding my brain. What if the chemo did not work? What if the tumor was still there? What if it did not shrink? What if I have to have more chemo? What if I have to have radiation? What if there is no surgical solution? What if the spots on my liver are still there? What if there are more? What if there are spots in my brain? What if there are new tumors somewhere else inside my body? What if they can do nothing about anything? What if none of this works? What if cancer is something I will have to manage for the rest of my life?

When I least expected it — reading, showering, lying in bed at 2 a.m. unable to sleep — these thoughts lazily filtered past my flimsy defenses like spaghetti through the holes of a colander. They danced around my bed like the white shadowy ghouls of the early days of cartoons, tall dancing specters, doing their creepy wavy dance with gaping dark mouths, taunting and teasing, spooky scary skeletons. Turning my mind off from these thoughts was impossible. Believe me, I tried. A lot. Since they will never go away, I have had to figure out how to live with them and not let them overtake my life.

As a list person, I use that methodical way of working through just about everything I do. That included getting through cancer. If I wanted to sleep ever again, I would have to work my way through my scary list. I needed to reassure myself that I had an emotional handle on the situation.

Decades of research and clinical trials and real-world application have proven that chemo will work in so many cases. Will I be one of those cases? I sure hope so. I have given myself the best advantages I can: top-notch doctors and a strong body through which they can do their work. I have to trust Dr. Jacobs, and I have to take the drugs. I am strong, and that tumor was small, weak, and doomed.

· · · · ·

Recovering from chemo proved to be an interesting process, mentally and physically. Six weeks post-chemo placed me squarely within the timeframe where I should see some actual recovery happening. Daily I was hitting up Ella and Alice for advice; I probably asked more questions about this phase than any other part of the process.

This round of treatment might be over, but chemo was not. Having chemotherapy is not like taking regular prescription drugs that have a short half-life inside the body. It takes several months before the drugs *start* to leave the system. Dr. Jacobs said it can take up to a year for many of the side effects to subside and to see normal blood work again. Other side effects such as nerve damage (neuropathy) can persist for years after treatments end.

For the three months of my treatments, the drugs were circulating, undiluted, through my body. Every week, even between my infusions, nurses drew my blood. This gave the doctor a sense of how the drugs were affecting my body. Using blood tests, the oncology team would determine if I was strong enough to face the next round. Sometimes, the infusion nurses were at odds with Dr. Jacobs' determination to continue, but as the captain, he always had the last word on the matter.

Each round was two weeks long: three days of infusion, 11 days to rest. The drugs were swimming around in my system nearly as potent on day 14 as they were on day one. The start of the next infusion just added to the amount of drugs inside of me. During the week between infusions, I could rest and endure the lingering side effects. I did not *recover* or *get over* the drugs. In 12 weeks, I received six doses of compounding medications, which is why by the sixth and final round I was reeling from fatigue that left me practically paralyzed, acid reflux that made every sleeping position in bed unbearable, and hands that looked like I was involved in a laboratory acid spill. With each round, the side effects got worse. I did my best to cope, and Louis tried to make life as normal as possible for me. I altered my life around the side effects, my new reality.

The only way to get over chemo is with time. And that time varies for everyone depending on their body and their chemotherapy drugs. In my case, I could expect to feel some relief at the four-week mark. At which point, the recovery presented as little things: my appetite was returning, the mouth sores were healing, my bleeding gums had subsided, my bloody noses were slowing down, my energy was coming back, and I saw the numbers on the scale creep up again. With each treatment, I lost ground with my weight, so it was no surprise that by the last treatment, I was back down to my lowest post-op weight.

I risked sounding ungrateful or petulant by trying to use my blog to explain this period. I was not giving the readers what they expected to see. Although chemotherapy was over, I was not celebrating. I expected I would be ready to dance in the streets when I was told I was cancer free. And even then, I could not imagine how it would feel to celebrate. I had been living a life full of uncertainties. What would it feel like to have good news? I spent too much energy explaining when I should have just focused on recovering.

My physical recovery turned out to be the easy part. By having the ability to return to my yoga practice, hiking, and running routines, I could measure my red blood cell recovery with relatively accurate predictions ahead of my weekly CBC (Complete Blood Count). For several weeks after chemo, I still had difficulty hiking uphill, stopping often to catch my breath. Countless times, I would break down in tears right there on the trail. I was not used to this kind of exhaustion; before cancer, I was running the trails and doing 10 mile hikes with very little effort. As the days and weeks passed after chemo, I could feel the aerobic recovery happening. I was thrilled when I felt recovered enough in late-April to train for the Anna's Wish 5K Race happening in June.

I have been active my entire life. Feeling out of shape is foreign to me. I just do not experience those sensations. And even if I did, I would never let them persist. No one had to tell me to walk after surgery or remind me to stay active to aid in my recovery. More often, they had to remind me to do the opposite: "Please give it a couple of weeks after surgery before you do anything crazy."

Being able to turn the feeling of being out of breath into something positive is quite difficult. Even for me. But for people who are not used to exercising, this could be the point where they give up. They might think recovery is too hard and they do not have the discipline to work through the discomfort. I subscribe to the notion that exercise and fitness equal life, even more so now that I have experienced firsthand how important my physical fitness was to my recovery and tolerance of the chemotherapy drugs.

When I was in the hospital recovering from my surgery in December, I was told that I would be out of bed and walking 24 hours post-op. I never fought it. No whining, no crying, no complaining — I just did it. The nurse stood back, gave instructions, and watched me sit up and swing my legs over the edge of the bed by myself. It seemed impossible that just a few hours earlier, heavy sedation had been the only way I could cope with the pain.

I would *never* lie in bed and feel sorry for myself and invent mental roadblocks. I felt the deep instinctual drive to get up and move no matter how much it hurt. The alternative, to wallow in self-pity, was never an option.

Twenty-four hours after surgery, I got up and walked one lap of the ward just as Dr. Quilici said I would. A few hours later,

I decided I wanted to do it again. Louis got me out of bed and took me for another lap. Holding a pillow to support my new stoma, my shoulders aching from the free-floating air in my abdomen, I finished the loop. When we reached my room, though, I felt a mild panic. Somewhere, deep in my bones, the message was being transmitted: do not get back into that bed yet. My body wanted to be up and moving. The new stoma throbbed, and the giant incision tugged, but I was determined to walk one more lap. And so, we did. This second time, as we approached my room, I felt a deep fatigue setting in. When I got back into bed, I broke down into tears. This was the deepest exhaustion I have ever felt.

The next day, I woke up with twice the amount of energy of the day before. Without the nurse's prompting, I was out of bed — I completed three laps before breakfast. After lunch, I walked five more laps. Later that evening, as I was chipping away at an additional five laps, the nurses told me that 30 times around the ward equaled one mile. I would need to walk that mile before they discharged me. My only question to them was, "And what is the lap record?" At this, they laughed. They refused to tell me because they needed me to rest a little, too.

I credit that difficult second lap I did with Louis on the day after surgery for my quick recovery. And so, with that in mind, I pushed myself with the physical challenges even during chemo. When hiking on the flats, I would add a couple more hills. When I was doing yoga and things felt tough, I would challenge myself to go through a few more poses, a few more minutes. Each time I pushed myself, I found the next day I felt even better. I am no doctor or physical therapist, but I think there is a lot to be said about not stopping when things are easy. One more lap. One more step. *Don't stop moving.*

I learned that recovering after surgery was not about lying around and taking it easy or complaining about how awful I felt. It was about tucking that stuff in the back drawer, getting up and walking. I would walk until I felt tired, then go just a little further. If I asked nothing of my body, it would never repair or get stronger. I just had to remember that I can do almost anything if I put my mind to it. Taking care of my body when I was healthy ensured that it was prepared for this major trauma. My body was ready and up to the task.

And that important reminder came when I needed it the most. A text from my yoga teacher while I was in the hospital recovering read: "*this* is what you've been practicing for."

· · · · ·

At the end of *The Lord of the Rings*, Frodo and the Hobbits turn for home after saving the world. This adventure takes close to six months for them to complete. It was full of outrageous situations and fantastic creatures which no one would believe if Frodo had not written it all down. The characters, like us, are immersed in the stress and excitement of the journey to destroy the Ring.

A less talented writer would have ended the book as Aragorn took his rightful throne. But JRR Tolkien continued the story through to the end of Frodo's life. He explores the weird drop in energy when we head for home after a long road trip. That feeling of being let down when returning to a normal life following an unbelievable adventure. We all recognize it, we all identify with it, and we have all experienced it.

Ringing the bell at the end of chemo, I felt like Frodo heading back to the Shire. The grand adventure was over. I was returning to a life I did not quite remember how to live. Would Bill Ferny be waiting for me, too? I was too tired to waste energy imagining twists to my story. Like Frodo, I was just hoping I could sit on my porch and watch a few sunsets in peace.

UNREMARKABLE

One of the most stressful stretches of time during this whole misadventure was the three weeks between the last day of chemo and the next PET scan. This was not a scan to see *if* I have a disease, or *if* I have something to worry about. This was a scan to find out *if* my treatment worked and *if* I was going to live. A lot of emotional weight to carry on my slumped and exhausted shoulders.

I know I can be a little too sunny sometimes. I am often reminded to control my enthusiasm. But I still felt confident that the tumor deep within my pelvis, binding my rectum to my vagina, was gone. With no scientific basis for this, I just had a *feeling* it was no longer there. When chemotherapy ended, I noticed that the chronic back pain I had been feeling prior to my diagnosis was gone. I could start packing on the pounds more easily and was having no problem holding on to them. My energy level was coming back up. Colleagues commented on how I sounded like myself again on phone calls and looked more like myself in video conferences. I felt better than I had on our anniversary the previous June. It was a relief on so many levels.

The day before the dreaded PET scan, Alice's words, colored with her wonderful Brooklyn accent, came over the phone loud and clear. "There is no way someone with a body full of cancer would have the energy that you have." Her warm laughter filled my ear. I had just rattled off a list of irrational fears to her and she had knocked each one back with the skill of Venus Williams. I knew she was right because I had lived it: when I was full of cancer, I was empty of energy.

Truthfully, I was the most worried about my liver. The first PET in November had revealed three tumors on it, and one showed hypermetabolic activity. My pre-scan anxieties were focused on that organ. Would all three metastases still be there after all that chemo? Dr. Jacobs had said that we were going to ignore the spots on my liver and just proceed with the chemotherapy. I held on to this non-action plan as proof that he expected the drugs to attack those spots as well. With chemo flooding every cell of my body, there was no way those tumors could avoid the poison. Just as I visualized the tumor on my rectum dissolving, I also imagined the tumors on my liver smoking and boiling away as the drugs filtered through the organ.

Even if someone can prove that visualization will not work in a clinical sense, I would find the results of that study irrelevant. Because what it did for my head was worth more than any research paper disproving its effectiveness. When I could not sleep, I would hold my hand over my liver and *direct* the chemo to attack the metastases. I always refused to believe that I was just a helpless witness to my amelioration.

I had to wait three weeks between my last infusion and the much-anticipated PET/CT scan — a lot of time to make myself ill with worry. It was difficult for both of us. I could see the concern on Louis' face when we talked about the upcoming scan. He said he was not worried about the results, but I know he was not delusional either.

Anticipating this PET scan was unlike any other scan, whether that be a mammogram and waiting for those results in the mail, or even the CT that first diagnosed this cancer. Though it seems unimaginable, worrying about a possible cancer diagnosis had been a lot easier to cope with than wondering how successful the chemotherapy had been.

I worked very hard to prevent my mind from wandering the dark dungeons of *Castle What-If* and to keep my thoughts on positive outcomes. To calm my mind, I would walk the dream tours of my little Victorian, stopping in each room to identify and address one fear at a time. Dr. Jacobs had predicted that the chemo would destroy the tumors. This could have happened. It was also possible that while the chemo wrought systemwide havoc, it destroyed the liver tumors as well. It seemed impossible that *new* cancer would grow or survive in the toxic environment created by chemotherapy, considering how thoroughly it wiped out my bone marrow.

Not wanting to scare myself, I kept my blog posts on the sunny side. Again, my theory was that if I wrote these optimistic posts, if *I* saw the words on the screen, I, too, might believe them, hold on to them, and give myself some much-needed reassurance. The amount of support that I received from readers was overwhelming. In fact, is there a word greater than overwhelming? *Crushing* has a negative connotation. But that would be a more accurate description of how it felt.

I awoke in the early hours of the morning on April 5, 2022, PET scan day. My chest felt heavy, the air thick and palpable. I was having difficulty drawing in a deep breath. Louis groggily asked me if everything was ok. I had bolted upright, waking him, too. "Can you feel it? Everyone is here with me."

It felt as if the entire world had taken a collective inhale and was holding their breath on my behalf. I have never felt anything so powerful. Suddenly, it all snapped into focus: I had never been alone in this fight. It seemed like everyone understood that this was bigger than anything that had come before. This PET scan would determine the course of the rest of my life.

Three weeks was a long time to wait to have the scan. As it worked out, I had to wait another week for the results. I learned early in this misadventure that people always relay bad news right away. Every hour that passed after the scan, the easier it became to breathe. It was possible, *no news is good news*, might be true this time.

I had done the hard mental work already, and I was ready to accept whatever was on those pages. No matter what the scan saw, we would deal with it. So, one week later, when Dr. Jacobs entered the exam room carrying the papers that contained my fate, I was serene.

Dr. Jacobs, however, was anything but serene. He launched straight into an explanation, line by line, of the two-page radiology report. That was the first thing I noticed: it was *only* two pages, and with very little writing on them. My first PET scan (the previous November) had been three pages, jammed full of scary words, metric measurements, complicated calculations, and confusing hypotheses. But this was *only* two pages?

My ears were ringing. I could hear him speaking in the far distance as he handed me the papers. The spots on my liver were gone. The tumor on my rectum was gone. The radiologist deemed the scan *unremarkable* except for a subtle thickening in the lower anterior pelvic region (Bill Ferny appears to have moved in while I was on my little chemo adventure). Dr. Quilici would schedule an exploratory surgery to get a visual.

I stared blankly at Dr. Jacobs as he continued to speak. I could not believe my ears. The chemo worked? The nightmarish 12 weeks that I had just been through were for something? He popped up out of his seat, his arms outstretched. "Congratulations!" He wrapped me in his arms, and I burst into tears on his shoulder.

This man had never once doubted these drugs would work. He made me believe anything was possible. His magic was real.

"You can keep the scan, by the way," he chuckled when he noticed I was tucking the papers into my purse.

"I didn't ask," I smirked. It felt good to laugh.

I held myself together through the elevator ride to the ground floor, but as soon as we stepped out onto the sunlit sidewalk of the medical campus, I simultaneously burst into tears and started laughing. I threw my arms out wide and flung myself at Louis, jumping up and down in his arms as he hugged me and lifted me off the ground. Sometimes good news passes through the doors of the Disney Cancer Center and pours out onto the sidewalk.

Science is incredible. My will to survive amazed even me. The power of the mind, body, spirit and collective energy of (literally) thousands of people was real and vital to my success.

The scan said my insides were unremarkable. Could there be anything more special than that?

· · · · ·

For the first time in months, I was feeling light and unburdened. The next surgery on May 5 would give Dr. Quilici a better view of what the PET scan had revealed and allow him to assess the viability of reversing my colostomy. I was looking forward to getting Dr. Quilici's take on the situation inside my pelvis. I was not so keen on the bowel cleanse I had to do the day before. My excitement at having confirmation of the success of chemo helped me get through those 36 hours of prep.

I met with Dr. Quilici in the days before my surgery. He reminded me that there was no guarantee he would reverse the colostomy, and I needed to keep an open mind about the outcome. There was a good chance that the cancer damaged my rectum beyond reconnection and repair. There was also a high probability that the *thickening* showed by the new scan would be remnants of the cancer. This was how the whole diagnosis process had begun months before. Both discoveries might mean I would not have the reversal. I told him I understood; I was ok with whatever he decided was best, and I believed I meant it. I was just grateful to be alive. A few short months ago, no one expected me to be here to ponder these scenarios at all.

I admit, though, when I awoke in the recovery room after surgery, reached under my blanket, and felt the ostomy appliance still stuck to me, I felt a rush of sadness and disappointment. *Oh well*, I thought. *This is just a minor inconvenience.* I trust Dr. Quilici, so if he left the colostomy in place, then I knew he had his reasons.

"It's not what you think." Louis kept stride with the gurney down the hall to my recovery room. Even through my anesthesia cloud, I could see that he was looking optimistic. I could not wait to hear the full story when Dr. Quilici came up to my room to debrief us.

We learned two bits of positive information from this surgery: the tumor was gone, and my rectum was healthy enough for a reversal. In fact, Dr. Quilici told me that if living with the colostomy was unbearable, he would keep me overnight and do the surgery in the morning. Recovery from that surgery, though, would mean delaying the start of the next round of treatments by several weeks.

He had found what he called *implants* — numerous, small cancerous deposits, called micro-metastases, that broke away from the primary tumor — in the area where the PET scan had detected the *subtle thickening*. Although it would have been possible to remove the ones he saw, where there are some, there are always more he cannot see. He left them alone, since radiation would be the most likely follow-up and everything within its field would be destroyed.

Dr. Quilici recommended that I not opt for the reversal, as the radiation would only damage the delicate healing tissue. Radiation comes with the side effect of severe diarrhea. I would have an easier time dealing with that, and the inevitable burns, if the colostomy remained in place. Since I had already experienced the benefit of having the colostomy during chemo, it was easy to agree with him. I would rather keep the colostomy during radiation as well.

My positivity had worked against me. I should have paid better attention to Ella and Alice, and everyone I know who has been through cancer. They all spent anywhere between nine months to a year in active treatment, tried several types of adjuvant treatments, and had multiple surgeries. No one who had any experience with this sort of thing expected me to beat colon cancer with one surgery and one round of chemo. I should have better prepared myself for another set of treatments. That was all on me.

Although, maybe there is something to be said about my tendency not to think too far ahead and to never expect bad news. Believing chemo would work, and not lifting my eyes to spend any energy worrying about radiation at the top of the hill, might have been an unexpected gift.

While recovering at home, I did not feel like posting on social media or blogging or answering texts or emails or entertaining phone calls from people wanting updates. Everyone was excited about the reversal and interested in hearing the results of the pathology, but I needed privacy to digest the information. I needed time to wrap my brain around the fact that my treatments were not over. A new dark cloud of uncertainty was looming in my future. I had to deal with this away from everyone, inside my head and out of sight. Slowly coming to grips with the outcome of the surgery, I did not need to do any part of my dark grieving in public.

In those first days following surgery, I was an emotional mess: deflated and disappointed. It seemed like the end was so close, all I had to do was reach out and grab it. I was desperate for this thing to be over. I wanted to wake up from surgery and then, against all odds, go on with my life as if nothing had ever happened. It felt as if someone had moved the finish line further away. The Universe pranking me because it noticed how badly I wanted it.

When I was 9 years old, Cabbage Patch Kids were all the rage. I wanted one in the worst way; I was practically frenzied. Christmas morning, my child radar saw a box shaped like the ones the dolls came packaged in. I ignored all the other gifts around the tree and went straight for it. When I tore off the paper, I discovered it was not a Cabbage Patch Kid at all. It was some other doll, a fancy old-fashioned thing, with a lacy dress and curly silk hair. Child Lisa may have tossed it aside, but clearly, I never forgot about it since I am still talking about it nearly four decades later.

That's how I felt about the outcome of my surgery.

I could have driven myself crazy thinking about all the possibilities, scenarios, and other things that I am not qualified to theorize about. My one consolation was to permit myself to feel deep disappointment, to mourn, rage, and sigh in exasperation for a few days. As long as that was not where my head lived the majority of the time, I could allow myself to feel those things once in a while. I had to remind myself: until we talked to Dr. Jacobs, we knew nothing about what was happening next. Until then, there was no point in expending more energy on the negative than was necessary to satisfy this compulsion.

I was unsure of what to do with myself between surgery and this appointment. I was restless. Regardless of how *good* I was feeling, I was recovering from abdominal surgery and was supposed to rest and heal with minimal activity for a few days. I was antsy and anxious and found it hard to sit still. Of course, the moment I moved too fast or pushed myself too hard, the fresh incisions spoke up and reminded me I was still healing and needed to relax. It seems like I should have learned from all those weeks of chemotherapy that resting and relaxing was not just my job; it was critical. I had to come up with ways to enjoy doing nothing.

Apparently, I learned nothing.

·　　·　　·　　·　　·

Having a doctor who sees me, and who appears to care genuinely about my outcome, made all the difference to my mental well-being. From the moment I met him, I felt that Dr. Jacobs took a personal interest in my health and maybe was even a little fond of me.

He walked into the exam room that Tuesday morning after my surgery and came straight for me. He grabbed both my hands in his and launched straight into the explanation of my new situation. "The chemo worked exactly as we expected it to." He was still holding my hands as he sat down across from me. "And you are doing even better at this point than I could have hoped."

Little known fact: every type of cancer affects our hearing. No one warned me about this. I had to find this out on my own. I could not hear my doctor's voice quite as well as the nurses' whispers in the hallway or the whir of the air conditioning unit on the roof of the building across the street. I could not hear the ends of sentences, regardless of whether the beginnings were reassuring or scary. Beyond Dr. Jacobs' exclamation when he entered the room, I heard nothing more during this discussion. This is why it was of vital importance that Louis was with me at every appointment. Thankfully, he heard everything and relayed it all to me in the car on the way home.

At this appointment, Dr. Jacobs only told us good news: the tumor was gone, and the small implants were all that remained of it. Radiation would finish them off. We also learned that when Dr. Quilici operated in December, he could not even access the rectal tumor because the cancer had essentially sealed off that part of my pelvis; when he operated this time, he described my pelvis as being *open*.

Dr. Jacobs would squeeze my hand in punctuation, his only tool available with which to bring me back into the conversation. I imagine my eyes were swirling black and white hypnotic spirals above my face mask, and he wanted to make sure he was getting through to me.

I was going to be referred to a radiation oncologist named Dr. Menzel because he would best understand how to approach my case. Unless I misunderstood Dr. Jacobs' explanation of my pathology all these months, every bit of cancer within my pelvis was colon cancer, regardless of where it was growing. The most obvious example was the tumor on my ovary — it was not ovarian cancer; it was colon cancer. The same is true of the tumor that had been on my rectum — it was not rectal cancer; it was colon cancer. Come to think of it, I had noticed that no one ever called it colorectal cancer. They always referred to it as colon cancer. It was all coming into focus now.

Dr. Jacobs gave my hand a few more reassuring squeezes. "This is all wonderful news." He concluded the appointment with his now customary hug and walked us out to the front desk.

"I've never seen him so giddy," Louis said while we waited for the elevator.

Despite all the positivity of the appointment, I had a meltdown during the drive home. The amount of stress and distress that had been my constant companion since November burst through the dam. I had not fully appreciated just how serious my situation had been until this morning. Blissful ignorance may have allowed me to endure the chemo, but now I was paying the price.

He let me cry it out, holding my hand while he drove. He waited for a lull in my sobs before speaking. "You've done nothing but fight and listen to everyone's advice and do what you were supposed to do. You did something incredible." During a break between my tears, he said, "Don't underestimate just how amazing this whole situation is."

I was crying so intensely I could barely breathe. "It was so scary," I wailed. "I've never been so scared in my whole life!"

He kissed my hand. "Who wouldn't be?"

HOPE

The little white moths that flit around the yard during the summer months captivated me when I was a child. Trying to catch one was an all-consuming obsession that could occupy my mind for hours if given the chance. I never, ever tried to snatch them while they were flying; I found it more fun to watch them flutter along their erratic path and try to guess where they would land.

I would follow one throughout the yard, waiting for it to settle so I could carefully collect it between my hands. I would open my little palms and watch my delicate prize walk around on my skin. While flying around, they look like they are nothing more than white paper wings. Getting an up-close look at them, they were like any other moth or butterfly with curious antennae; large, complicated insect eyes; furry bodies; and delicate legs. It amazed me that something so tiny could be so perfect. They sparked my curiosity about the world of flying insects.

It seemed like such an exceptional accomplishment to catch one. This skill has followed me into adulthood. I am an expert at catching wayward moths who find their way into our house.

When I spot a familiar white paper moth in the yard now, I have a hard time resisting the urge to follow and catch it. When I give in, the reward is just as sweet as when I was young.

For me, *hope* during chemotherapy was a little white moth dancing into view. Even though I had no business hoping that the chemo would work perfectly, I believed it would. I would have quiet moments when I would become giddy and think *I'm going to be ok.* I did not want to be disappointed, and yet, I could not resist chasing it every time hope fluttered into my line of sight.

Chasing *hope* during cancer treatments required the same patience and delicate touch as chasing those white moths. I did not want to smush or injure the little moth; I did not want to squelch my delicate hope either.

It was ok to feel the allure of *hope*, carefully catch it, and hold it in my hand for a little while.

PART FOUR

"We are stardust, we are golden, we are billion-year-old carbon,
and we've got to get ourselves back to the garden."
– Joni Mitchell

MAGIC CANCER

"No, a Geiger counter cannot detect radiation coming off your body," Dr. Paul Menzel, my new Radiation Oncologist said. "A lot of patients ask about that." Too bad. I had a Geiger counter in my Amazon cart, its purchase pending his answer to my burning question.

I was looking forward to radiation like a rocket launch. It was exciting to know a giant machine with a cure rested on the horizon. "This will all begin within the next two weeks," Dr. Menzel said. It seemed fitting that the youngest doctor on my team would oversee the most science fiction treatment. His offices were on the ground floor of the Disney Cancer Center.

I admit I was excited to get this ball rolling. Preparing for radiation, the next powerful weapon against *The Abdominable*, had predictable logistical steps: PET scan, surgery, consult, CT scan, and a planning session that involved body measurements taken with fancy computers and calculated with high-level math, and body mapping with tattoos. There was even a rumor that lasers were involved. I was disappointed to find out light bulbs would not strobe on and off when I walked past them.

Twelve weeks would elapse between the end of chemo and the beginning of radiation — the same amount of time I had had chemo, I now went with no treatment. I tried to remain calm, but on the inside, I was terrified that the cancer was growing unchecked. "This is one of the most difficult periods," my Aunt Lorraine commiserated.

I spent many sleepless nights worrying about the unknown and every waking moment avoiding research on radiation and its side effects. Exhausted from relaxing, all I wanted was to feel useful and productive. I had hoped to slip back into some activities that made me feel like myself again. I would have to sit out the upcoming summer concert season, but I could start meeting up with some friends one-on-one. They were cautious and always wore their masks around me. It was amazing how receiving a hug from those friends I had not seen since before cancer could send me into hysterical tears. I think I may have unnerved at least one of them with the intensity of my reaction, but I did not care.

"I couldn't have done any of this without you," I said to Ella. This was the first time I could thank her in person. It had been over six months since I had last seen her. My face in her hair, her familiar scent enveloped me. I could not hold on to her tightly enough, and she reciprocated. She had been a lifeline through all this, all accomplished entirely through texts, emails, and phone calls. She was the conduit through which I poured my gratitude to Lori and Alice, who lived too far away for me to hug.

So many friends who had supported me from afar — calling and texting almost daily, sending food and gifts, and emailing photos and videos of their dogs and children — were now in my world as tangible humans once again. For so many months, life was going on without me. Cancer would consign seeing friends to a memory, and all I would ever have of them would be words and images on my iPad screen.

The delay in the start of radiation also allowed me to try my hand at going places other than the hospital, doctor's office, or the treatment center. I dipped my toes back into an echo of my former daily life, unencumbered by crushing fatigue and oppressive side effects.

It felt great to burn off some of the energy that seemed to build exponentially in my muscles. As the post-chemo weeks passed, my legs became twitchy and restless at night. Coupled with the lingering neuropathy in my feet, this made it difficult to sleep. I found incredible joy in training for the upcoming race even if I would not break any personal speed records. Pam was happy to take me hiking and pass a few afternoons playing cello duets in her living room.

Despite my enthusiasm, I had to stop running and hiking at the end of May when I developed a mysterious limp and stiffness in my ankles that made it difficult to negotiate uneven terrain; it hurt to take the step down into our sunken living room, where our pianos were. I also developed pain in my left shoulder and my thumbs making it uncomfortable to play my cello.

We brought these fresh pains to Dr. Jacobs right away. His explanation was lucid and consoling: joint pain is a common delayed effect of chemotherapy, often appearing several weeks after treatment has ended. My Aunt Lorraine's experience was echoing in my ears: chemotherapy triggered her dormant rheumatoid arthritis. I shoved that thought out of my brain. RA was the last thing I needed on top of everything else. Ella developed food allergies after chemotherapy. That did not happen to me, though I certainly had several new food aversions.

Over the next few weeks, my systems gradually regulated themselves, the limp disappeared, and I could get back on the trails and resume training for the race. Though my shoulder continued to hurt for several more months, being able to practice yoga was making me feel strong and centered, while the more aerobic activities burned off all that extra energy accumulating in my muscles. It felt great being back to my old — I have extra energy to burn — self.

Not that I enjoyed being bald, I just appreciated that it made it obvious to strangers that something was wrong with me. Hair growth came with many unexpected and strange feelings attached. My cancer treatments not yet finished, the world needed to know I was still in this thing. I toyed with shaving my hair to the scalp again just to prolong that feeling during radiation. Ironic how I resisted shaving my head during chemo, and now I was resisting growing my hair back. As I stared longingly at the bald patients in the waiting room, I came to understand why it had been so easy for me to recognize recovering Cancer Club members out in the wild.

The longer I had to wait to start radiation, the more my mind explored the darker corners of this whole situation. Nurse Negative Nancy's short life expectancy prediction and the 10% survival rate were duking it out for the winner of *The Scariest Information of 2022 Award*.

Louis confided that when I received my diagnosis in December 2021, the doctors and nurses gave him the impression that I would not live to see the end of 2022. Certainly, if I had had no treatments, that would have been the case. I never asked Dr. Jacobs for my prognosis. He would have given me the real numbers and settled this score. Without his verdict, I could remain blissfully ignorant of how close I came to losing this fight before it even began.

Because I had such dark and thoroughly ingrained reactions to the notion of chemotherapy in the past, Lori and Pam worried I would refuse to take it. I would receive texts from them telling me that life was worth the fight. They were right: I had to overcome gobs of anxiety and fear before accepting these life-saving drugs into my body. Meditating on the reality that I had no choice allowed me to dig deep to find the courage and strength to face it. I was lucky to receive the message from the Universe "Accept chemotherapy into your body as your ally, and you will be healed." From that moment on, I was a changed person, ready to begin the treatment.

An even darker mystery kept me up at night: how long was that cancer growing inside me before I started having symptoms? I did not go from perfectly healthy to aggressive Stage-4C Colon Cancer overnight. Was the ovarian cyst the previous summer the first sign of something going dreadfully wrong, or was it just a coincidence? I was still reeling from how quickly things spiraled out of control in just a couple of months.

What if Dr. Quilici had not come into my life? What if I had put up with Dr. Unger's lack of communication for another week or two? How close was my bowel to rupturing? And if it had, would there have been the proper care available to get me through it or would I have succumbed to sepsis?

I was not quiet about my discomfort during those months. I was unrelenting in trying to find answers. It was a pointless exercise to explore the *what if's?* I had done everything necessary to solve the mystery, even if I took a few bad turns along the way.

I have heard so many stories of (especially) elderly women who hid their obvious cancer symptoms from their families because of embarrassment, while others were ignorant of what the symptoms could mean. Even worse, some must have known something terrible was going on, but chose not to face it. If they never talk to the doctor, they will never have the test that confirms their worst fear.

I knew something was wrong. Even if I did not know precisely what it was, I knew it was deadly serious. Every cell in my body was transmitting the distress signal, and I had two choices: listen or ignore. I chose not to ignore the alarm bells when the cancer was brewing. I do not plan on doing that ever in the future.

I have heard plenty of positive stories from people who survived colon cancer. Alice's recovery is a testament to the multitude of colon cancer treatments available, and to the success of the variations. Although her kidneys shut down while on Oxaliplatin infusions, radiation and an oral chemotherapy drug worked for her. A ten-year survivor, she is on the road to proving Nurse Negative Nancy wrong. She has given me untold amounts of strength and support through this. I draw so much inspiration from her and she keeps me going when times get rough.

Not all stories have happy endings, though. The father of one of Andrew's closest friends since the second grade, had endured a year of treatments. He beat his colon cancer, only to fall victim to a complication during his colostomy reversal surgery. Just when it seemed like he was going to move on with his life, he was gone. In the wake of this sudden loss, there was an 8-year-old boy without a father and a young widow. A decade later, I am living the same situation, and haunted by this turn of events.

How could stories like this not affect me while going through the same thing? I know that treatments for colon cancer are highly successful nowadays. Still, I cannot help thinking about him. Yes, we are all going to die at some point, but no one wants to do it this young. And we certainly do not want to think we will overcome cancer only to die from a surgical mistake.

I tried very hard not to fixate on my hypothetical prognosis. For all I know, the doctors were expecting me to snuff it within a couple of weeks. It never occurred to me I would experience anything but a full recovery. I would not call it willful ignorance; I just saw, in the greater arc of my life, cancer as a blip. Looking ahead, a year seems like a massive amount of time to pass. But every December we act amazed at how fast the new year has flown by.

This lost year of my life passed in a chemical haze.

Knowing that I was going to have chemo rattled me. But, knowing I was going to be fighting for my life made me more determined. I never doubted a full recovery awaited me at the end of the road. I owe this confidence, not arrogance, to *never* asking, "How long do I have to live?"

The weeks passed after chemo. I spent much of that time tamping down worries about the cancer re-growing while I was off treatment and waiting for radiation to start. It seemed reasonable to wonder, "If chemo is over, can the cancer grow again?" No one seemed to rush me into the next phase of treatment. Dr. Jacobs had been pushy about getting the PET scan done right away after chemo and shuffling me into surgery as soon as possible. But after that surgery, everyone, Dr. Jacobs included, seemed pretty laid back. He never gave the impression that we were on a tight schedule and needed to hurry into radiation treatments.

I still saw Dr. Jacobs every two weeks for blood tests and a basic physical. At each of these visits, he would always ask about the lingering and late effects I was experiencing. The most serious ones were gone, but dry skin, cold sensitivity in my hands, tingling in the soles of my feet, numb toes, and the occasional recurrence of the strange metallic taste stuck around for months. I already knew that those side effects, along with the random appearance of other late effects, could last for up to a year after treatments ended. Facing down radiation with oral chemo meant that the clock counting down that year was about to be reset.

Louis constantly reminded me to trust the Grown Ups — they wanted me to spend this time relaxing. So, I spent those long weeks using the dry skin on my hands as a visual reminder that the drugs had done the same thing to the cancer. The cancer cannot grow and spread and do more damage if the 5-FU gave me severe dry and peeling skin that could not heal in 12 weeks. I had to believe that the remaining tumor implants were just as damaged.

Swinging between unbridled optimism and crippling fear was dangerous to my emotional state. This was not the time to fall apart; it was time to wear my positive thoughts as a delicate crown of wildflowers and to ride my grey pony in a cloud of white moths and hummingbirds.

My only job was to keep my eye on the prize. Before radiation began, I needed to eat and put on a few more pounds, exercise to get my body back in shape, and to get my head back in the game and on my team. If Dr. Jacobs and Dr. Menzel were not talking about uncertain outcomes, then there was no point in me fabricating frightening scenarios in my head at 2:30 in the morning.

The interminable timeline leading up to radiation stretched ahead of me. It was a lot to ask of me to remain patient for twelve weeks. When I complained about the delay, a friend responded, "We call this 'hurry up and wait' in the military."

Weeks earlier, Jeremy, my college friend who was diagnosed with non-Hodgkin's lymphoma, had texted, "It's a heavy burden being a young cancer survivor." His words rang louder than ever in my head as I lay in the CT scanner during my radiation planning session. One week ahead of my first radiation treatment, this CT was just to calibrate the machine, in no way a diagnostic test. Still, I feared the images on the screen in the control room would reveal my body riddled with new tumors. It was becoming clear that this would be part of my burden: forever living with the anxiety of what might grow, regrow, mutate, and devour the inside of my body.

Jeremy called me the day before radiation began. We have known each other since we were 18. Although we may not see each other as often as we would like, he still holds the power to make me laugh until I can barely breathe. As we roared like teenagers over the phone that afternoon, I felt that burden lessening with each howl and shriek. Although his burden differs from mine, we both needed a break from the future. He gave me an unexpected and beautiful gift that day on the phone.

During chemotherapy, I leaned heavily on my survivor friends. Alice reminded me that I was not crazy and that what I was going through was not unique or worrisome. Mouth sores suck, but Amanda had had them, too, and told me, "You'll get through this." The fatigue could be overwhelming and frightening, but Ella encouraged me, "You will feel better tomorrow." And, every time I started to panic or despair, Louis had me repeat back to him the mantra: "Fear the cancer, not the chemo."

I did not want to let anyone else's chemo experience sabotage my delicate courage; I needed to experience the drugs on my own terms. It proved more interesting and helpful to compare our experiences *after* my regimen was complete.

But radiation seemed so concrete, so straightforward and scientific, that I felt emboldened to ask about their experiences ahead of my first treatment. It's like asking, "How did it feel when you walked across the hot coals?" It hurts, and it burns because heat is a constant. The stories I was hearing about radiation did not scare me, they just helped me steel myself against what was coming. They were not telling me the worst parts, and I was thankful for that. When this was over, I would have a unique tale to tell. I did not know what would happen during radiation until I was in it, just like I did not know before chemo started. But how different could my experience be from theirs? This time, I would not be at the mercy of liquid chemistry. I was about to be hit full force with solid physics[15].

· · · · ·

Another unexpected side effect of cancer is the inability to accept good news. From April to June, from all the doctors at all the appointments, I only heard good things, positive things, encouraging things, miraculous things; and yet, I did not seem capable of accepting them. It seems reasonable to assume a cancer patient would latch on furiously with both hands to any news that even remotely smacked of positivity. Turns out, it does not work like that.

My dear Suzy texted me the day after her post-chemo PET to tell me that her scan seemed promising. But before I could finish typing my response, another text appeared, "I don't think I can take this news at face value." She spent the next few

---

[15] I never took physics in high school, so I have no idea what I'm talking about.

minutes listing all the reasons she thought this scan was inaccurate and why every single ache, pain, and sensation in her body signaled more cancer that the scan did not pick up. She was speaking aloud the words that I had been thinking to myself all these weeks: the scans must be wrong, and I have the definitive proof of why.

Old cancer. New cancer. Hidden cancer. Magic cancer. Undiscovered cancer. Unnamed cancer. Confounding cancer. Incurable cancer. One of these has to be inside my body.

Suzy confirmed I was not alone in these fears. We spent many afternoons talking about this; it was like talking with myself. It was frightening how similar our feelings were on the subject.

No one should ever say to a person with cancer, "Don't worry, everything will be ok." *Nothing* is ever ok. *No one* can predict the future. We need reassurance that we are not crazy, and we are not alone. We must believe that it is ok to not be ok.

Ella and I had a long lunch where we could speak about our experiences in person. In 2020, she passed the 10-year remission mark, and yet, I could see and hear that the emotions surrounding her cancer diagnosis were just as raw and real as they were on day one. Nothing has changed. Over a decade has passed, and she is still saying the same things that Suzy and I were saying mere weeks after our chemotherapies had ended.

I heard these same sentiments from parents of children who survived childhood and infant cancers. As unlikely as it seems, two of my college friends each had a child who had cancer diagnoses before the age of 5. Their children survived and have been living normal lives, post-treatment, for many years. And yet, they tell me they find it impossible to shake the disbelief that their children are healthy.

Parents focus intense energy on their precious children, which gives them the superhuman strength to get through this unimaginable thing. They have to keep a clear head to process the information in the face of the ultimate horror. To figure out a way to present the situation to a small child who may not know what is going on, is a heroic undertaking. As that child grows, asks questions, and becomes more cognizant of the situation, those parents face additional stresses at each screening. How does a parent accept good news at face value when the life of their child is hanging in the balance? How do they not transmit that fear to the child year after year?

Doctors Quilici, Jacobs, and Menzel each asked me to repeat back to them the situation *as you understand it to be,* several times between my surgery in May and the start of radiation in June. No one corrected me, so I took this as a sign that I had grasped the important concepts involved. Obviously, the doctors wanted to make sure that I was aware of what was going on before they cut, drugged, and irradiated me. I had Louis there to confirm or correct me on our drives home from all appointments. But I am an adult, not a child or an uncertain teenager. I am aware of my situation even if I wallow in disbelief and indulge in a little self-pity from time to time. The real danger was not that I would not understand what was happening to me, but that I would do too much research and scare myself.

Many blog readers wrongly assumed that the addition of radiation to my treatment plan was a surprise to me. I may have been disappointed, but I was not delusional. I think the opposite was closer to the truth: everyone else assumed I was cancer-free, and *they* were the ones caught off-guard by the news of radiation. Whatever their rationale, now they saw it as their job to convince me that going along with radiation was the best course of action. They bombarded me with their own justifications, which only overloaded my systems. Deciding to undergo a different cancer treatment is not like deciding between taking cough medicine or a cough drop. There is no option, choice, or debate. Because I trust my oncologist completely, there was no other option than to follow his plan. My only question when each new treatment plan was presented was, "When do you need me to show up?"

I may have found out the hard way, but with cancer, it is no surprise to find out there will have to be more treatments, more drugs, more scans, more everything. Wellness is the more difficult concept to understand. So, in a weird turn of events, I put in a lot of effort correcting everyone: I know I still have cancer and I never questioned whether to do radiation. I appreciated everyone's enthusiasm for a miracle cure after one round of chemo, but obviously, that is an unrealistic expectation with Stage-4C cancer, even if they did not want to see it.

Some believed that radiation was *insurance* that the cancer does not come back. Just like chemotherapy, there is a lot of misunderstanding about what radiation does. It is another form of cancer treatment that exacts collateral damage on the body to kill the cancer cells. Chemotherapy poisons the water supply; radiation comes in after to carpet bomb the area.

Radiation is a 120-year-old sci-fi treatment to remove whatever is left of the cancer. Even if it did not show up on the PET scan, there was still some cancer inside of me. Intensity-Modulated Radiation Therapy (IMRT) targets and damages the tumor's DNA, which stops the cancer cells from dividing and growing, stunting tumor growth. Most times, radiation even kills the cancer cells. When I was inside the machine, I imagined those little remaining implants burning and smoking and exploding, just as during chemo I visualized the tumor shriveling and dissolving.

I understood the excitement surrounding how well the chemotherapy had worked. And I was excited, too. But my treatment was not over. I needed to fight and fight until I was cancer-free. And that news had not come yet. No one needed to whisper the word *cancer* around me, and they did not need to pretend there was no more cancer inside me, either.

A few hours after my radiation planning session, Louis and I were watching television. Nothing out of the ordinary was happening, but he could see I was on the verge of tears. Of course, it only took him asking, "What's on your mind?" for me to burst out sobbing. He gathered me up in his arms, stroking the new baby soft hair on my head.

"What the doctors are saying is good news, right? I'm not misunderstanding them?"

"Yes, it is all good news. Tell me what you think you heard them say."

I took a deep breath and spewed the list of unbelievable facts between sobs. "Dr. Quilici saw the tumor was gone. Dr. Jacobs said the PET showed the liver metastases are gone. Dr. Menzel said these little things left behind are going to be burned away with the radiation."

Louis just kept reminding me that none of them were worried at that point. All the doctors had this under control and my only job was to follow directions. I had to try very hard not to inject any unnecessary anxiety into this thing. "It's ok to be happy about this."

Just like during chemo, I was crying for no good reason. Again, panicking over imagined fears. I knew from experience that once this storm passed, the clouds in my head would clear. My tears subsided, and I could feel the superficial layer of muddy uncertainty washing away, revealing tiny seeds of courage. I could see it clearly now: radiation was also going to bring large amounts of emotional turmoil, and I needed to prepare my delicate new garden for the oncoming deluge.

But right now, it was safe to open my hand and see that the tiny white moth crawling around on my palm was real.

CHEMO BRAIN

I needed to relearn how to trust my sense of reality. How quickly I forgot that chemo made my brain cloudy and confused. I lost touch with reality on more than one occasion. For all I know I was out to lunch the entire time I was on the drugs. How could I trust my perception? Louis was constantly reminding me of things that had happened during the weeks that I was on chemo. How was it possible that I had absolutely no memory of them?

Louis tells a story from my third infusion. One evening while we were watching tv, I walked away and never came back. Realizing I had been gone longer than expected, he found me in the bathroom, sitting on the toilet naked, and crying. I was inconsolable. "Oh no, what's the matter?" He knelt in front of the toilet while I leaned against him and sobbed. The 5-FU pump was hanging from the towel rack next to me and my clothes were in a pile by the bathtub. It was possible that I had simply lost my mind. I can hear him through the distant fog of the memory repeating "Oh sweet thing…" He let me cry until I was out of tears. His voice is the only thing I remember of the incident.

The steroids that they gave me in combination with my chemotherapy drugs added their own unique brand of side effects to the mix. *Roid Rage,* which we traditionally associate with bodybuilders, was a scary side effect for me. It struck me hard during the 3rd infusion, halfway through my treatments. I believe Louis has protected me from more episodes than the one I remember, which is a kindness on his part.

One night, I screamed at the top of my lungs at Louis. My memory does not include whatever happened leading up to this that made me believe this was an appropriate response. I remember standing in the kitchen, gripping the center island in both hands, and screaming at him. I can see his stunned face through the cloud of this memory. We have never had any disagreements when we even raised our voices, much less one of us been driven to screaming. I can feel the rage of that moment and taste the harsh tears. What saddens me the most is the look on his face; his expression of surprise and hurt will be burned into my memory forever. There were so many things that happened during chemo that I wish I had not forgotten, but I would give anything to forget this. He knew it was the steroids causing me to behave that way. Still, this was a shitty way to repay him for all the care and love he had selflessly given.

Being out of touch with reality was not pleasant, funny, or entertaining. It was very frightening. Dr. Jacobs had to remind me, more than once, that the drugs had left me with fractured memory. "You just don't remember how bad it was, but we do," he said, tipping his head toward Louis. It had been nearly a year since my diagnosis, and I was trying to convince him that "chemo wasn't all that bad." His laughter rang more with relief than amusement.

Without Louis or my journals, I would have had very little proof of what chemotherapy was really like. Revisiting certain entries, no matter how much I strained, I had no recollection of writing them. The things I had said or felt bewildered and fascinated me. There are large chunks of time that I cannot account for, and others that come back to me like a fever dream. I had to rely on Louis to fill in the gaps in my memory.

Chemo brain was not a funny T-shirt slogan. It was more than trailing off during a sentence, the inability to find the right word, or being unable to complete a thought. Large swathes of time disappeared much the same way as being in the operating room, receiving the first sedatives, then finding myself awake in the recovery room.

On a lighter note, one evening I got up from the sofa and walked with purpose to the kitchen. Standing at the center island, I held up a water bottle like I had just won an Academy Award. As if I were continuing a conversation I had been having in my head, I said, "You know, the thing is…"

Louis stared at me expectantly, the uncomfortable long pause dragging on. "What's the thing?" he asked. He strained to get my attention from the other room.

"Huh?" I blinked at him. "What's what thing?"

Although we laughed and I shrugged it off with good humor, part of me was a little horrified by the whole incident. We still joke about the weird stuff I did during chemo, but we also know they were anything but a joke.

At a pace even slower than my new hair growth, I hardly noticed the changes were happening. Yet I was rising out of the murky depths of the drugs. Clear-headed and lucid, I was about to begin my radiation treatments. I had every reason to believe the words coming out of my mouth, yet I was still questioning my perception at every turn. It prevented me from entirely accepting this new reality filled with good things.

The question I have now is how long will this disbelief last? Looking at all the cancer survivors that I know, I think the answer to that question is forever.

JACK-IN-THE-BOX

Knowing how obsessed I was becoming with the new hummingbird nest beside my patio, my friend Miriam sent me a wonderful gift to pass the time during radiation: hand feeders. Impossible though it seems, coaxing a hummingbird to eat out of a person's hand can be done. Miriam was one hundred percent certain that if anyone could do it, it was me.

At the very least, she had created a monster. She tapped into the obsessive side of my personality that endeavors to be great at everything I attempt. That includes wrangling wild birds. I believed I could do this thing.

Night after night, while the June heat was burning off, and the sun was setting, I sat patiently in the rocking chair on our patio with the small hand feeders perched on my knees. A sign of the changing of the air creature guard, the first bats of the evening flitted through the yard. The last of the chattering hummingbirds spent those waning minutes of twilight getting in their last sips of my homemade nectar from the hanging feeders above my head. The very first evening I tried this, one bird came close enough to get a good look at the new little feeders I had introduced into his world. I knew it was only a matter of time before I charmed him into eating out of my hand.

Hummingbirds exist on a different frequency than we do. We must seem like elephants to them, slow and plodding. Their entire universe is wrapped up in the quarter acre of our yard; they eat, sleep, and breed within our trees year after year, waging their little hummingbird wars over the best food sources and mates. They harm nothing, waste nothing, and cause no destruction. We could learn a lot from them, and all animals, if we slow down even more and learn to be present in our own lives.

During those weeks, I practiced being wholly present with my dogs. While I was reading on the patio, oblivious to the world around me, Luna would bring me back by jumping on the sofa and demanding to be petted. I learned to give in to her, close the book and set it aside so I could be completely present with her at that moment.

"I am petting Luna," I would think to myself, and petting the scruffy dog became the most beautiful activity to be doing. Every time, she reacted to the shift in my intention. One of those rare dogs that purrs, she would coo and grumble, pressing her forehead into my side, and flashing her best puppy eyes at me. Being with her like this became a daily meditation.

At first, it was difficult for me to accept that relaxing was an acceptable way to pass the time. Although it took some time, I could give in and allow this to become a way of life for me. My days settled into a comfortable routine which, I admit, I would not be as eager to give up as I thought I would be. A little (big) part of me mourned that this leisurely way of life would soon end with the start of IMRT.

At my first consultation, Dr. Menzel and his assistant, Cindy, talked me through the expected side effects of IMRT and when to recognize the signs that it was imperative that I reach out to them. With their years of experience, they knew what I was headed for, but never gave me a reason to be afraid. They started by warning me about the least scary side effect: fatigue. We wanted to know why this happens. We could understand why drugs would cause it, but why would radiation have that effect? Dr. Menzel said that no one really knows why, just that it is a near certainty it will. Cindy commented that the routine of making the drive to the office through the I-5 traffic every day would give anyone deep fatigue.

Dr. Menzel prescribed me 29 radiation treatments. The first 25 would hit a wide zone, covering my entire abdomen, 360 degrees, from the bottom of my sternum to my pelvic bone. The final four treatments, called boosters, would only hit 10% of that initial area, focusing on the location of the original tumor in my lower pelvis, but would employ a stronger dose of X-rays.

Unlike localized radiation treatments for certain other types of cancers, my radiation would be extensive, affecting the entire abdomen and cooking all my organs. Although every attempt would be made to avoid certain delicate tissues with the radiation, my entire digestive tract was in the line of fire. At the very least, diarrhea would be unavoidable. It was highly likely that it would become so severe that I would need medical intervention. I was feeling cocky and overly confident, so I barely paid attention to what they were saying. For the most part, I had sailed through chemotherapy without major stomach or intestinal problems. I was convinced that radiation would be the same. They could save this information for someone who needs it.

Dr. Jacobs prescribed an oral chemotherapy drug called Xeloda (Capecitabine) to go along with radiation. This was the same drug that Alice took after her reaction to the infused chemotherapy drugs; she could answer my questions about what to expect. As I understood it, the drug enhances the effects of the IMRT by sensitizing cells, both cancerous and healthy, to the radiation treatment. This meant that they could give me a larger quantity of zaps at a lower daily dose of radiation. The major drawback was that it would also enhance the side effects of radiation.

I had to laugh at myself for being nervous about taking the new pills, considering the massive chemotherapy I endured just a couple of months earlier. What was I so afraid of? Xeloda was the same drug as 5-FU, just in pill form. Unfortunately, while we were watching for Hand and Foot Syndrome to return, we were blind to another more serious side effect taking root in the background.

Radiation began with little fanfare. I climbed onto the table in the machine; the nurses adjusted the table according to the tattoo dots given to me during the planning session; the machine made some clicky noises while it spun around me three times, and then *voilà! Medium rare Lisa is served.* It took less than 10 minutes from start to finish — aligning my new tattoos with the array of lasers shooting out of the walls and ceiling took longer than the treatment itself.

I was feeling good, just a little more tired than usual. For the first three weeks of treatments, I did not experience any major side effects aside from growing fatigue and mild nausea. Overall, I was doing well, and although everyone around me seemed pleased, I noticed that the nurses seemed to look at me a bit sideways. Like they were listening to the slowing music and wondering after which note the jack-in-the-box would pop out.

During those early consultations and treatments, most of the questions focused on appetite, colostomy output, and pain levels. Every Friday, I met with Dr. Menzel and Cindy to talk about how I was doing. Though they seemed cautiously optimistic, they remained lucid with their warnings. The refrain week after week: "If anything changes, call us right away." Paulette, my radiation nurse, issued a sober warning when I seemed a little too confident for her liking. "When things go bad with radiation, it happens fast. You won't question whether or not you need to call."

Radiation is invisible. I could not see it, touch it, or feel it. When people looked at me, I looked normal. There were no outward signs that I was having it. When the machine was bombarding me with rays, I felt nothing. But clearly radiation was doing something to my body because the effects were real. And they were about to turn deadly serious.

During the first week of treatments, I experienced dizziness and nausea moments after climbing out of the machine. Everyone seemed a little concerned. Paulette suggested I might be motion sick from laying inside the machine and watching it go around me. I started taking Zofran again (I had plenty of the anti-nausea medication leftover from chemo) an hour before every treatment and that helped. Thankfully, there was an even simpler solution: I kept my eyes closed during treatments. Like magic, the dizziness was under control.

The nutritionist set me on five small meals per day, made up of low fiber, high carbohydrates. The expectation was that I would not overburden my inflamed digestive tract and that I could maintain my hard-earned weight gain. In those first weeks of treatment, I maintained my weight, my appetite not much affected by the treatments. I was feeling pretty darn good about my ability to heed Dr. Quilici's warning: "If she doesn't eat, none of this will work."

Radiation fatigue is real. Even after experiencing it, I still cannot possibly explain it. I would wake up in the morning feeling normal; I would practice yoga or go for a hike. At 12:45 p.m. I would climb into the machine feeling just fine. When the treatment was complete, I would limp clumsily back to the waiting room a changed person. Sitting in the lobby, I waited for the woozy feelings to pass before walking to the car. I could drive myself to the first seven treatments. But as Paulette had predicted, there was no question when driving by myself was no longer possible.

Around the 10th treatment, because of the soaring summer temperatures, I was told to stop all strenuous outdoor activities. Even though I still felt strong, my core was inflamed, and I was losing my ability to regulate my internal temperature; I was at risk of overheating. Though at first, I complained like an insolent teenager, of course I listened to Paulette and stopped hiking and running. She had years of experience, so she knew what she was talking about. Soon after, I even reached a point where I found it impossible to tolerate sunlight. I was rapidly overheating on the short walk from the car to the cancer center door.

Around the halfway point of treatments, number 15, there appeared a sensation in my core similar to having done a hard abdominal workout. My muscles felt weak and tired. At first, I thought nothing of it. I assumed that by replacing hiking with more yoga, I had overworked my abdominal muscles. This feeling continued to increase over the next two days, so I mentioned it to Paulette.

"Remember," Paulette said as she adjusted me in the machine, "this isn't like chemo, where you had two week breaks between doses. Radiation happens daily, and you get no chance to recover. Each day is worse than the one before. Your last week is going to be the hardest." Paulette, always the straight-shooter, had made it crystal clear that I was on a slow march toward the worst days of my life. I just did not want to hear it.

One afternoon after treatment, the *tired* abdominal sensations switched to actual pain. I may have overreacted a touch, since it was very reminiscent of the intestinal pain I was feeling prior to my diagnosis. Post-traumatic stress in cancer patients is real, so my level of panic escalated rapidly. Clearly, this was not an intestinal problem — I was not nauseous, gassy, or having diarrhea. It was an intense, radiating, all-encompassing, and cramping pain that overtook my entire body. Ibuprofen did not dull the pain, so I spent the night writhing in bed. Louis could no longer disguise his panic. Around 3 a.m., he asked if I thought he should take me to the emergency room. It got that bad.

One great thing about my doctors, all my doctors, is that they spring to action swiftly, compassionately, and decisively at the first sign of distress. I called Dr. Menzel's office the next morning, telling Cindy I did not want to have my treatment that day until I could see him. She had no problem fixing the schedule and hurrying me into an exam room.

I liked that Dr. Menzel did not play fast and loose with pain medications. He told me frequently he avoids taking pills until he absolutely has to. I was glad we saw eye-to-eye on this. Before cancer, I rarely took even so much as an aspirin for a headache. Here I was now: a walking pharmacy. I did not want a handful of pills to mask my problems. I wanted actual solutions. I was so thankful to have had a doctor who understood this.

While I was explaining the pain to him, he made it immediately clear that this was an expected reaction. It was reassuring to learn that nothing terrible was happening to me and, most importantly, that I was not unique. Turns out that the same fitness that saved my life after surgery and during chemo was now working against me during radiation. Without a layer of fat in my abdomen to diffuse and filter the radiation as it passed through to my organs, my muscles were getting a full blast of the rays. They were becoming burnt and irritated and spasming in reaction.

Dr. Menzel did not want to prescribe an opiate for the pain, which I was glad to hear because, outside of coping with post-surgical pain, I prefer to stay away from those medications. Instead, he prescribed an antispasmodic which, as he expected, gave me some relief.

Thankfully, he also allowed me to take the day off from treatment. We all hoped that I could recover enough over the weekend before resuming. It was easy to postpone a treatment. If, at any point during the rest of the treatments, I needed to, I could ask to take a break. There are no heroes in radiation.

Because it was the Fourth of July weekend, I ended up having a four-day vacation from treatment. It felt great to have the long weekend to recover. My appetite was coming back, and renewed energy coursed through me. Facing the upcoming week of radiation did not seem as daunting. I went into the next four rounds with a positive attitude and fresh resolve.

In a direct challenge to my stubbornness, they had warned me that Xeloda, combined with the IMRT, would give me diarrhea. Dr. Quilici had been very clear about this being the main reason he left my colostomy in place ahead of radiation. Until treatments were over, it would be easier to deal with this side effect. I have learned an important lesson: when Dr. Quilici speaks, listen closely. Eventually, I would develop second-degree burns at the base of my tailbone, which, by the end of treatments, turned into third-degree burns covering the entire area between my buttocks. I could not imagine trying to endure unrelenting diarrhea with those burns in my butt crack.

With just seven treatments to go, the diarrhea that everyone had been warning me about appeared. It was violent and unrelenting. I was taking an entire box of Imodium (Loperamide) every 24 hours, which only held the diarrhea at bay until it wore off, then it was back in full force. I began dropping weight rapidly. In three short days, I lost five precious pounds. Everyone saw this coming except me. I could no longer afford to keep my eyes squeezed shut and my fingers plunged deep into my ears.

There are many obvious benefits of being fit and healthy. But one unexpected benefit is that it was crystal clear to my doctors when I was not feeling well. When I am healthy, they see me with varying levels of high energy: I walk fast, sit up straight, am garrulous and inquisitive, make eye contact, and am always engaged in every interaction. Any slight change in those behaviors means they can recognize something is wrong. With one look at me, they can see that I do not feel well. Unfortunately, if someone is normally low energy and often comes to the office complaining that they are not feeling well, it could be difficult for their doctor to appreciate how bad their situation is when it really matters.

Louis joked he could tell my energy was returning after chemo by how talkative [read: grumpy and argumentative] I was in the mornings. The nurses in the oncology department could tell how I was feeling based on how quickly I made the walk down the long hall to the scale.

Dr. Jacobs was alarmed when he saw me moments after my 23rd radiation treatment: my blood pressure had fallen to a worrisome level. Low blood pressure is a dangerous side effect of the Xeloda. This was the first hint that I was headed for a serious reaction. He toyed with giving me IV fluids that afternoon, but we held off. I was so exhausted. I just wanted to get home and lie down.

I made it through treatment the next afternoon but paid a heavy price. Pam had driven me to that treatment. She could see that I was not doing well. She had been sharing driving duties with Louis during my treatments all these weeks. Having accompanied me to so many previous appointments and witnessing the immediate side effects of the IMRT, she knew what to expect. But this was different. She had never seen me come out of the machine looking and acting as downtrodden as I did that day. On the car ride home, I was uncharacteristically quiet and was visibly struggling with the pain. She was right to be worried. The rest of the afternoon, I had zero energy and was struggling with renewed abdominal pain and unrelenting diarrhea. I knew I did not feel well, but nothing could prepare me for what was coming.

The next morning, there was no mistaking that things were not going right inside of me. I was sitting on the sofa watching tv, unable to stomach the flour biscuits I had made to eat with my morning dose of Xeloda. I felt like I was sinking backward into my head. My hearing became fuzzy, my vision tunneled, and I could feel my insides shaking. I was woozy and weak. All I wanted to do was lay down and sleep. My lizard brain was screaming to find a rock under which to curl up.

Louis took my blood pressure multiple times to make sure the reading was correct; he even did a few measurements on himself to test that the machine was not faulty. We could not believe what we were seeing: my blood pressure was 70/52.

The jack had popped out of the box.

WILTED FLOWER

When chemotherapy started, they gave us a poster to hang on our refrigerator outlining the different side effects and when to call either Dr. Jacobs' office or 9-1-1. We never thought we would need this chart during radiation. We had already taken it down. My mind lingered on this poster. I believed we had jinxed this whole thing with that one simple act.

Louis called Dr. Jacobs' office and, of course, they told us to come in right away. Every time Louis spoke, he sounded distant. My eyelids felt heavy, and I was drowsy. The pain in my abdomen continued to flare up, making me even more miserable. I could not stop the tears and I worried I could not hold myself together once we reached the office.

Everyone in the oncology department had jumped to action before we arrived; they were already waiting for us. We did not even need to check in. They had posted a nurse in the waiting area for me. I never appreciated how long the hallway was to reach Dr. Jacobs' exam area. Like a horror movie where our hero is trying to run, but a camera trick stretches the hall into an inconceivable distance. I thought I would never reach the scale. With every wobbly step, I clung to Louis for stability and support, frustrated tears stinging my eyes. I wondered if I had enough energy to finish the walk on my own two feet.

This was the first time, during all my treatments, through all my surgeries, and in the seven months since my diagnosis, that I felt genuine fear.

I was taken to an exam room, Dr. Jacobs hot on our heels. The first thing he did was take my hand and reassure me he was going to take care of me. Even during chemo, feeling my crappiest, I still had the energy to talk and joke and be as normal as one could be on heavy drugs. This time, I was not talking. I did not feel well. Tears were leaking uncontrollably. I went deep inside, disinterested in speaking or taking part in the real world. Even in the presence of my beloved oncologist, I could not bring myself to respond to his questions with anything more than one-syllable grunts and moans. Louis had to do all the translating.

Dr. Jacobs had me lie down so he could palpate my abdomen. I was certain that all this excitement proved that the cancer was worse. It had finally happened: something new and untreatable had appeared. Today, I expected everything to start over again from the beginning. He tried to help me sit up, then thought better of it when he realized he was the one doing all the work. He instructed a nurse to get me a blanket so I could lie there while they made arrangements with the infusion center. Dr. Jacobs gave my furry head a gentle rub, reassured Louis one more time that I would be better soon, and then declared in an indignant tone that I was now off the Xeloda. The little boy with the broken arm would have been impressed with Dr. Jacobs' transformation: I had just watched my favorite teddy bear reveal himself to have been a grizzly all along.

All I could do was lay there, eyes closed, and unmoving. Maybe if I kept perfectly still, cancer could not find me under the thin white blanket. Within minutes, Nurse Debbie showed up with a wheelchair to take me to the infusion center to receive intravenous hydration. Climbing into the wheelchair felt like admitting defeat. I am tough, but I am not Wonder Woman. "You're making me so sad," she cooed, resting her hand lightly on my shoulder. "You look like a wilted flower. But don't worry, once you get fluids, you'll perk up and be your usual sunny self again." I was so lucky that so many people felt invested in my well-being.

In the infusion center, I was back in the care of Nurses Terry and Abby. This time the volume turned way up on encouragement. Terry kept reassuring me I would feel better faster than I imagined. She hung a bag of lactated ringers and one of Zofran on the IV tree and then inserted a needle into my portacath with her expert touch. I had not had time to apply the lidocaine numbing cream ahead of time, so it was crucial that the nurse was sure-handed and confident in her ability to keep the pain to a minimum. Accessing the port is not a pleasant procedure.

About 15 minutes after the saline began flowing into me, Terry added a push of Dexamethasone (steroid), which perked me up almost instantly. The colors of the hills outside my window became more saturated, the room became brighter, and it felt like my neck could hold my head up again. The infusion lasted two hours. I spent most of that time staring out the window, watching people waiting for the elevators in Dr. Quilici's building across the campus. I was rising out of the muck, and my fear was slowly melting away.

Since this was a Friday, and everyone wanted me to survive the weekend unsupervised, they postponed my radiation treatment for the day to Monday. With only five treatments remaining of the 29 prescribed, all the nurses kept reassuring me I was well past the important part of the treatment. I had now ventured into the *we-just-want-to-be-sure-it's-really-gone* stage. Everything from here on out was just bonus treatments. It was alright if I needed to stop.

Whoa whoa whoa. Who said anything about stopping? I am the type of person who wants to finish an assigned task all the way to the end. I signed up for a marathon; I was not going to stop at 26 miles.

Despite my fear, it was important to step back in my panic and trust in the knowledge, experience, and confidence of my doctors and nurses to support me through it. Once again, I was handing myself over to the Team of Grown Ups and they expected me to trust them unquestioningly. That day, we witnessed a different side of everyone in the oncology department. When the shit came down, everyone was cool, calculating, reassuring, and focused. Even though I was frightened out of my mind, their calm demeanor during this episode was supernatural. I was the delicate white moth fluttering weakly in their careful hands.

We went home, ready to face the weekend, coated in a thin layer of courage. Although I had no reason to feel this way, I was sure I would have a good weekend and, of course, this would be the last hydration infusion I would need. Naturally, my intestines had other plans. Sunday evening, the loperamide stopped working. I found no reprieve from the diarrhea. Anything I drank or ate came through my system untouched. Exhausted from emptying my colostomy bag every few minutes, the walk back and forth to the bathroom was becoming more difficult to endure with each trip. My strength drained from me. I felt deep despair.

"Please, don't make me do this anymore." Radiation had reduced me to begging and sobbing. "Can you call them?" I could barely breathe.

Louis never faltered. "No." He was quiet but firm. "You're going to finish. We all know you can do it. They'll take care of you." There was no stopping the tears and panic. The room was spinning. I felt myself slipping into that thick cocoon that protects my brain from having to cope with the scary stuff. No question about it, we would need to call Dr. Jacobs in the morning. I expected to have to repeat the hydration infusion.

Something strange happened inside my head. Even though just moments before I had begged to end the treatments altogether, the thought of having to put off even one more radiation treatment filled me with annoyance. I liked that my treatments would end on a Friday. If I had to postpone one more time, then I would not be ending until the following Monday. That did not align with my sense of squares and straight lines. No matter what, I wanted to finish this week on time and on schedule. I could dig deep and if it meant satisfying my obsessive side to get through this, then so be it. Whatever it takes to round out the calendar.

Louis could not drive me that Monday morning, so Andrew was up to bat. He could not help much during my radiation treatments because he had been back east visiting his grandparents for a month. Now, he was ready to take charge and take care of Mom. I think every parent can relate to how I felt on that car ride, not wanting to worry him while he navigated the early morning rush hour traffic. I had to hold on to him for support as we walked from the car to the cancer center, but I knew he was learning an important lesson about parents being human.

Arriving at the office, I was worse than I was on Friday. Barely able to put one foot in front of the other, Nurse Brian cradled me close to him for support down the epically long hall. "I should have brought a wheelchair," he muttered. He waved to another nurse at the end of the hall, directing her to find one.

"No," I sniffled, "I *have* to walk." After what felt like an epic journey, we arrived at the scale. My detached legs struggled with the low step up. I had lost seven pounds in four days. As I stood there, yellow liquid poured out of my stoma and into the bag. I could not control my tears, either.

"It's ok. We've got you now." Brian brought me to an exam room. The doctor was right behind us and again took my hand while he spoke to me.

"You're going to have hydration every day before each treatment until the end." Dr. Jacobs was sympathetic and cool. "You just have to get through this. You'll feel better after this week, I promise." Within minutes, a wheelchair arrived, and Brian was pushing me back toward the infusion center. I felt deflated. This was the second time in four days that I had to be wheeled into the infusion center. Andrew had the honor of pushing me the rest of the way to my favorite corner cubicle. The nurses were already busy preparing my IV tree.

Again, the mix of hydration and medications brought me out of my stupor. The world was coming back into bright focus. Beyond my privacy curtain, I could hear Terry on the phone with the radiation department, letting them know I was back in their care and questioning whether Dr. Menzel wanted me to have my treatment that day or not. When faced with the possibility of another pause in my IMRT, I felt more determined than ever to plow forward. I would not back down now. This may even get dangerous. I had been warned. But I saw no other choice. I had only finished the first 26 miles of this marathon;

less than a quarter mile was all that stood between me and the rest of my life.

Lori's voice echoed in my cloudy brain, "I can do hard things." And it appeared this upcoming week would be the hardest of all *the things*.

"What are you doing here?" It surprised Paulette to see me two hours later when I walked into the radiation department for my 25th treatment.

"I'm doing it." I stood up as straight as I could in a lame attempt to fool her into thinking that I looked normal. She said she did not feel comfortable giving me the treatment until she spoke with Dr. Menzel herself. Of course, he gave his approval, but he had to see me when I was done with this treatment. This would be the last of the extensive area IMRT; tomorrow I would begin the booster doses. After today, my abdominal muscles and many of my internal organs could begin healing. Days earlier, I had asked Cindy how the booster doses would differ from the first 25 treatments. Her hesitation implied that the next four days would be no picnic. Radiation treatments had so far exceeded my expectations, and the hard part had yet to begin.

After treatment, I was seen by Dr. Menzel and Cindy together. They reassured me that everything was under control. Both Dr. Jacobs and he would support me through these final four boosters. "We'll take good care of you." This was not the first time I had heard this reassurance. Everyone expected my blood pressure to come back up after I was off the Xeloda, and no matter how much diarrhea I experienced, they could support me with the IV infusions. I would be ok. I could do this. Together, we *all* could do this.

Altogether, I received six doses of IV hydration, every morning before radiation. The fluid infusions left me stronger and better able to face the boosters. Although the diarrhea did not stop, and my appetite was nonexistent, I was safe. The Grown Ups were in charge.

Paulette's words rang in my head all week, "When things go bad, it happens fast." She was absolutely right. My head was spinning from the dehydration. I developed new burns in the crease between my hips and thighs and on the exposed skin around my stoma, while the burns between my buttocks went from second-degree to third-degree with just one booster treatment. It was unbearable to sit, so I spent most of my time at home lying in repose like a Roman courtier. My portacath was sore from being accessed daily for the hydration treatments, and my abdominal muscles ached. I was uncomfortable getting into bed, walking around the house, wearing pants, sitting in the car. My lower abdomen was tanned and swollen. The IMRT had burnt my pubic hair off in a perfectly straight line, delineating the radiation area. The diarrhea continued full force, and I was going through one box of Imodium every day. My bladder was so irritated it burned to urinate; I was struggling with incontinence and running to the bathroom four or five times during the night to pee, making it difficult to get enough sleep.

On Friday, as I sat in the infusion center for what would be my sixth hydration treatment, I received a call from Dr. Menzel's office. The recommended booster dosage was between three and five treatments. He had settled on four because it was in the middle. It was now up to me to decide if I would receive the fourth treatment on this day. If I felt like I could not go on, he was comfortable ending at three.

I had contemplated this possibility the night before, during my multiple trips to the bathroom. What should I do if given the choice? Get the last treatment or stop? After all, Dr. Menzel had said three was good enough. With just one word, I could make this all stop. But the finish line was in sight; all I had to do was stretch out my chest and break through the tape.

I knew if I did not have this last treatment, I would spend the rest of my life wondering, "Did I give up too soon?" If the cancer reappeared in the next few years, I knew I would return to this moment and think, "Stupid girl, this wouldn't have happened if you had just done the final one." I wanted no regrets about anything to do with my treatments. I am the one who will have to spend the next several decades of my life living in the shadow of cancer. Why would I voluntarily give myself something concrete to worry about?

And so, I took that last treatment. I accepted the rays into this body, radiating hope and positivity back at the machine. My eyes closed tight as the machine spun around me for the last time. I listened as the horrible radioactive buzzing dove into the deep low frequencies of the booster treatments. I pictured myself 10, 20, 30 years down the line, looking back on this moment. I wanted to be proud of the young woman who had the courage to endure one more painful treatment because she had been filled with compassion for her future self.

Cindy gave me a *Certificate of Completion* and a hug. Louis took photos of me sitting outside the Disney Cancer Center. That night, as we climbed into bed, I broke down yet again. "I can't believe I did any of this."

"You did it with bravery, strength, and grace." Louis had become an expert at helping me ride the emotional waves.

Despite his certainty, I could not agree with him. I just had to wait a few weeks to feel meaningful healing, and nine weeks to get my act together before facing one more surgery. A future beyond that surgery awaited me. A life with no cancer, no questions, and a renewed appreciation for how precious living is.

One week after my last radiation treatment, I was back in Dr. Jacobs' office for my weekly physical and bloodwork. In contrast to the previous week, this time I walked from the waiting area to the scale unassisted. All the nurses cheered me on: "You look amazing!" "I can't believe it!" "You're incredible!" I saw it as an affirmation that I was not delusional. In just a few short days, I had bounced back to where the medical staff could celebrate the visible victory.

Dr. Jacobs burst through the exam room door. "Oh, thank goodness! I was so worried about you!" He pulled me in for a hug. Relief flooded through me. A lot had been riding on this outcome. Holding me at arm's length, he gently scolded, "You almost gave me a heart attack." I believed him.

My physical pointed to a full recovery on the near horizon. I just had to keep eating and hopefully, by the end of the week, I could wean off the Imodium. He palpated my abdomen, and we were both relieved that much of the sensitivity had already subsided. He prescribed as many calories as I could consume, lots of rest, and pampering. I could definitely do all that.

He handed out one more hug. "You're not allowed to feel bad ever again."

"Thank you, thank you, thank you," I kept repeating into his shoulder. I believe he possesses some sort of magic that can make that come true. Because I know that if he has anything to do with it, then that last week of radiation treatment will remain forever the worst I have ever felt in my life. From here on out, it can only get better.

LEAVES

Around the time that I was starting radiation treatments, I received a text from Suzy telling me she was beginning a second round of chemotherapy. We had been through our first round of chemotherapy together that spring. Now she was back in the infusion center for six more rounds of the drugs, this time without Oxaliplatin.

"The good news is I can have ice in my lemonade this summer!" Suzy rejoiced at that small, but very important, prize.

We made plans to meet up after our treatment one afternoon. We spent some time together in the courtyard of the cancer center, talking and hugging. She was hooked up to her 5-FU pump, and I was still dizzy from radiation. We had only known each other for a couple of weeks, yet we laughed like childhood friends. Other patients walked past and smiled at us. Cancer survivors do not need to be sad all the time. In fact, we may be some of the most joy-filled people alive.

Suzy grew quiet, lost in the breeze moving through the branches of a nearby tree. We were holding hands. More to herself than to me, she whispered, "The leaves are so beautiful."

There was peace in knowing the breeze would always blow through those trees, with or without us.

Several months earlier, I had been a hair's breadth away from death. Near-death experiences are not always filled with white lights and floating sensations. I had met Death, and this time, he had accepted my bargain. I came away from that encounter reborn as a new species. Though I survived to live among my family and friends again, I was more alone than ever as they tried to understand this new version of me. I perceived the world in a way that only those who have almost died can understand. The words to describe this world are not yet invented. This is why this instant kinship with Suzy transcends friendship.

We may have looked common, sitting on the bench, holding hands. But we were on another plane, standing together on a crumbling precipice, our toes dangling over the edge, facing our own doom. Holding on to each other meant survival. Our bond forged in starlight. Together, we could be both brave and vulnerable as we stared down the eyes of cancer.

Since last December, I had spent countless hours alone watching the breeze through the trees in our backyard, mesmerized by the shimmering leaves, a thousand hummingbirds, and the sunlight sparkling through the branches. The intense comfort of seeing Suzy's reaction to the leaves made my heart swell with affection for her. Sitting on a bench while the rest of the world rushed past, we quietly experienced the simplicity of the moment, the blue sky above, and the bright sunlight on our skin. We required no words. We did not have to invent frustrating platitudes about how precious life is. We understood how unfortunate it was that we had to look Death in the eye to learn this lesson.

All our thoughts seemed to be transmitted to each other through the language of the rustling leaves. It had been many long minutes since we had spoken aloud, yet the conversation had continued.

She had a sweet habit of petting my baby soft hair, one of my favorite signs of affection. Her gentle hand still caressing my head, she said, "I'm so glad we found each other."

THE HAWK AND THE CROW

One night, I dreamt of a hawk and a crow sitting on a rock. They stared deeply into each other's eyes. Transfixed, I could not look away. Bloodied and beaten up, they remained fierce and wondrous in their mystical beauty. With a sudden coordinated movement, they turned their heads and looked straight at me.

I woke with a gasp and a jolt, waking Louis with my sudden scare. "Did you have another nightmare?" Unlike the deep sleep filled with vibrant dreams I experienced during chemo, nightmares plagued me during radiation.

"No, nothing like that." He tried to collect me up into his arms so we could go back to sleep, but I waved him off. I sat up straight and checked my watch. "3:20 a.m. This is the third night in a row that I've woken up at this exact time." His interest now piqued, I described the dream, and he agreed, this was no nightmare.

That morning, needing an explanation of what the hawk and crow might symbolize, I surfed the web for *dream symbols* and *dream animals*. I would never find what I was looking for on the internet because none of the descriptions would ever apply to what I dreamed. It was all wrong. None of what I was reading made any sense. Louis had a distinct impression of this unsettling dream: it was a vision.

It would seem reasonable to expect that I would have dreams filled with many creatures. My life is full of animals: my dogs, the backyard menagerie of squirrels and skunks, baby raccoons, howling coyotes, hooting owls, the bouquet of hummingbirds, and my totem and friend: the Cooper's hawk. Crows also visit our yard — they sit on the telephone wire and cackle at the dogs, drop stolen peanuts from the trees, and watch me with interest as I toss cut-up apples into our grass for them to carry off. They have an otherworldly language that ranges from spooky gurgles and garbles that sound like mispronounced words, to resonant clicks and clucks as if they were playing claves in the trees. The crow is Louis' totem.

This was a dream in which both our totem birds appeared to me in striking realism. It would not carry any meaning found on the internet. I needed to ponder it thoughtfully. Whatever meaning I drew from it, therefore, would have to be unforced and, like the dream, reveal itself at an unexpected time. Now, just a few days past the end of radiation treatments, I had the time and energy to examine this dream. I meditated on the vision while I was on the yoga mat, allowed the birds to fly around inside my head while I was playing my cello, and looked to the real hawks and crows above for clues while I was hiking on the trails. No matter how the vision would begin, it always ended with a thrill as the two birds, beat up, but vibrantly alive, turned to look directly *at me.*

"This is all," words from a dark and prophetic chemo dream rang in my ears one morning while I was out hiking alone. I stopped in my tracks as the realization washed over me. The meaning was in front of me all along: Louis and me, *esto es todo.*

A powerful alliance. We had come through my cancer a stronger couple. Despite my breakdowns and tantrums, we never had a single real argument. We have never been one of those couples that constantly bickers and jabs. We are very fond of each other and amused by each other's quirks. We have always been affectionate and doting, and always are touching no matter where we are: holding hands in every elevator or leaning against each other while we wait in line at the grocery store. Even if we went to bed in a snit once in a while, we still cuddled up as if nothing was the matter.

The Age of Cancer was no different.

We often laugh at the Oscar Wilde quote: "A second marriage is the triumph of hope over experience." I came out aces; Louis ended up with the defective spouse.

By my count, we made at least one hundred trips between doctor appointments, various treatments, and multiple surgeries. On so many of those trips, I would glance over at Louis, trying to tamp down his anxiety in the driver's seat. I would think back to the early days when we were dating. Those exciting days when anything was possible with the new person in the front seat. Driving home from an appointment ahead of my surgery in September, I wondered out loud, "If, on our first date, you had seen the future and saw that this was going to happen, would you still have married me?"

"Silly girl!" he laughed. "First, that's a stupid question. And second, there's nothing they could have shown me to make me not want to marry you!"

In the first 13 years of our relationship, we faced nothing like this cancer diagnosis. We promised "in sickness and in health," but we never imagined this. Buying and selling houses is stressful and raising a blended family is challenging, but nothing compared to mustering our collective power to fight cancer.

Like the hawk and crow of my dream, each of us is powerful on our own. But together, we are unstoppable. Although we may not have come out of this experience unscathed, we are a fierce and fearsome team.

I was gifted with an open channel to strange realms during cancer. Helped along by the poisonous chemotherapy drugs being pumped into me, I lived during those 12 weeks on what I can only describe as another plane of existence. Before the diagnosis, I felt apart from others. Now, I could feel that I was *a part* of everything. I am not *outside* the life on this planet; I *am* the life on this planet. I am more than this body. I am stardust.

Watching the red-tail hawks swirl on thermals above the mountain while I hiked, I learned to quiet my mind so I could imagine what they saw from their vantage point. I meditated on what the tops of clouds looked like. I marveled that some trees rustled, even when there was not a perceptible breeze. I was open to all methods of healing. My body, mind, and spirit needed unique elements with which to do that.

Historically, I never put much credence in the ridiculousness that is crystal healing. I never had any interest in learning about the power of crystals. Once, I attended a class at a mystic store because I walked in on it accidentally. I stayed only because I knew it would look rude if I turned around and walked back out. Stones can heal? *Puh-leeze.* But thanks for the free bracelet.

While still recovering in the hospital after my diagnosis, I felt an inexplicable fascination with healing crystals. From my hospital bed, I purchased a small amethyst carved in the shape of Ganesh and a sodalite stone. I clutched these two stones, every hour of every day, through the entire 12 weeks of chemo.

At night, I held them over my pelvis and during the day I wore them around my neck in a little pouch. I did not care how stupid this all looked or sounded to anyone; I was all in with these silly stones. The amethyst would grow hot to the touch and become unbearable against my skin, so I figured something must be happening. I only stopped wearing the stones because I just sort of *wandered away* from them naturally. Two weeks after chemo had ended, I realized I had not been carrying them around. I figured there must be a deep reason I abandoned them on my nightstand untouched.

Louis theorized the stones had soaked up all the cancer and bad juju that they could hold, and I must have sensed that they no longer served a purpose. It was time to bury the stones and put this dark energy to rest. I decided that when I was cancer-free, I would take them up to the mountain and bury them off the trail.

Just before my PET scan in April, I opened the pouch to discover that Ganesh's ear had broken off. I considered this discovery for quite some time. I decided that this must symbolize that the cancer had left my body. I had solved the symbolic mystery and felt confident about the upcoming PET scan. I left the stones on my yoga altar until I was ready to bury them. I was glad I waited to bury them, because after my next surgery in September, I would come to the shocking realization of what the actual message of the broken stone had been.

Frequency (sound bath) healing was another thing I had outright dismissed in the past, so of course, I would try it now. I began listening to 528 Hz every night as I slept. The combination of white noise and complicated musical phrases encouraged me to find calmness and sometimes even quiet my mind completely. Even with the pump making noise when it injected the 5-FU drug into my body every 90 seconds, I could disengage from reality and fall asleep. Just like I learned to be present with the dogs, I learned to be present with sleeping. The frequency soundtrack became such a part of our nightly routine that Louis depended on it, too. He would often remind me to turn it on before we turned out the lights.

Honestly, I doubt the stones or the sound bath actually *did* anything other than comfort me. But is that not enough? I do not think there has to be scientific proof of something in order for it to work or have an actual effect. I also did not care what people thought about me using those things. They brought me comfort and peace during the worst period of my life, and that should be enough.

. . . . .

Jeremy's words continued to play in my mind. "It's a heavy burden, being a young cancer survivor." He so aptly articulated how I had been feeling. My obsession with deciphering the meaning for myself was overwhelming.

The act of *not* googling colon cancer survival rates early on was itself the answer that seemed to best reflect my reality. I would live with cancer for multiple decades of my life. I would have to learn to cope with this emotional burden, and not let it devour my happiness down the road.

If given the opportunity, would I want to know how long I had to live? This was an interesting game to play when I was healthy, with no shadows looming over me. Sometimes I thought I would want to know. Since having cancer, this exercise has taken on new meaning — my response to this question changing by the minute. Maybe it would be helpful to know how much time I have left so I could prepare and savor my remaining years. But right now, I do not want to know. I think life is much sweeter when I enjoy each moment as it comes, not knowing what awaits me around the corner.

I looked at my life in five-year chunks after accidentally reading that scary statistic. What if that were true and I only have five years left? Was I prepared to close up shop and return to stardust at 53? How will I celebrate that birthday, knowing that during that year the next scan, or the next test, could show that the cancer is back?

When I let my mind wander along those thoughts, something stronger rose from the depths: a little voice saying, "You're going to feel silly when you're 85 and you remember thinking these things." No one can predict my life expectancy. It will be better for my peace of mind to suppose my life will continue on like everyone else's, just like I had taken for granted before I had cancer.

As much as I could, I avoided using the words "this is unfair." Despite my best efforts, they swirled around in my head like a tornado. This whole situation was profoundly unfair. My whole life I have done all the right things: I am vegan and fit; I have never smoked, and I stopped using alcohol and caffeine; I avoid chemical household cleaners and Teflon coated frying pans; I make my own homemade deodorant, for fuck's sake. I am the exact type of person who is not supposed to get any sort of cancer, much less late-stage colon cancer at 47. If anyone had a right to stomp and scream "This is unfair!" it was me.

It was unavoidable that I would have some dark thoughts infiltrating my brain, which should have surprised no one. I thought of vile people who tortured children and mutilated animals. They could use a good dose of cancer. They spread violence throughout the world while in perfect health. *Why don't those monsters have cancer?* Some people tried to dissuade me from thinking this way, but I believed I was entitled to my anger.

I spent most of my time trying to prevent myself from descending into the murky swamp of bad thoughts, but sometimes I would dip my little toe in just to satisfy that part of me that needed to scream, "This is so outrageously unfair!" It was ok to indulge that side once in a while, as long as it did not overtake my delicate happiness and become the place where my head always lived.

It was always difficult to muster the courage to face the reality that I could be gone at any moment. Every day since my diagnosis was an *extra* day of my life. I am living in my own afterlife. Another heavy burden.

I had heard stories about people for whom it seemed treatments were working, only for them to take a sudden and mortal turn. Would I be one of those people? I had already survived through the summer. Would something happen before Thanksgiving? Would I live to see another birthday next spring? What news would the next PET scan bring?

I took stock of my daily life during those 10 months of treatment. Turned out, all the things I used to think were so important were not. I have suffered from chronic insomnia my whole life. Surprisingly, I sleep better with cancer than I ever had before.

I came to the frustrating conclusion that I had not accomplished so many of the things I had expected to do by this age. A career full of starts and stops, I had never experienced long-term job stability. Before I met Louis and moved to Los Angeles, I had never been married, nor lived in one place, longer than ten years. I wanted to survive long enough to live out this love affair with Louis. We deserved to grow old together. It did not seem fair that now, when my life was becoming something I had always wanted, it would be taken away. Because it wasn't fair.

I had no choice but to give in. When I finally said the words *"this is so unfair"* out loud, it felt as if a dam had burst. The relief was powerful.

I was doing well enough that Louis trusted me to go hiking alone. He understood I needed the solitude. "It *is* unfair," my inner voice boomed in my head, drowning out the sound of my shoes on the sandy trail. I was struggling to hold myself together, the pressure in my chest building as I became overwhelmed with the reality of it all. I clumsily stepped off the trail, crashing through the tall grasses, and scaring a small rabbit who had been hiding. Sitting down on a boulder with a clear view overlooking the San Fernando Valley, I said aloud, "This is *sooooo* unfair." Fully expecting the rocks and scrub brush to agree with me, I looked around. They gave no sign they had even heard me.

Above me was a crisp blue, Southern California sky, without a single cloud. A blue scrub jay called "chuk-chuk-chuk" from somewhere in the bushes behind me. I barely breathed, listening to all the layers of noises made by scurrying lizards in the dirt, birds hopping between low branches, and the distant din of the traffic below.

It was all *so fucking unfair.* And yet, here I was alive and hiking after all that chemo and radiation. Other than the cancer, nothing else was wrong with me. What was I complaining about?

I received the message loud and clear. A breeze rustled a nearby tree. I watched the shimmering leaves. A sense of peace came over me.

I had cheated Death this one time. *We will have a bargain from now on; someday you get to have me. But not today. I demand more time.*

I picked myself up and made my way back to the trail, filled with a renewed sense of purpose. *When I'm done with this thing, I won't be the same person.* I knew this deep in my cells, and I could already feel the shift happening. There is nothing tragic about the fact that all things must end. It is only a tragedy if I am delusional enough to think that I am going to be the one person who lives forever. The crime was in missing out on the opportunity to be absolutely alive.

The months pressed on, treatments progressed, and I had nothing *but* time to contemplate my life. I would break down in tears on my yoga mat, hug my knees in close, and whisper, "Thank you, Body, for saving me." My language was a direct reflection of my attitude toward living a long life. I used words like *when* and *someday* and never said *if* or *hopefully.* Chemo would work. Radiation would work. *When* this is over, I *am* going to hike the Trans Catalina Trail. We *will* celebrate our 20th anniversary. I *am* going to see Andrew get grey hair.

There was never a doubt in my mind that treatment would be successful. I could feel the cancer dissolving; I could feel my body repairing. After each treatment, I could feel the changes that healing brought with it. One small step at a time, in three-month increments, I came back to myself.

Cancer was one hell of a *twist* to my life. I had no plans to waste this opportunity for rebirth.

NICE TRY, CANCER

Another hummingbird in a nest, memories of radiation, just like chemotherapy, blended into the half-light of my peripheral vision. It seemed so impossible that something so dramatic could lose its significance. Like so many other experiences, it was a fading dream to look back on with curiosity and fascination. The burns healed, new pink skin replacing the blackened areas, and it became difficult to remember just how serious they had been. Though the skin of my lower abdomen remained tanned from the radiation for many weeks, it would fade back to my natural color. I no longer had abdominal pain, and my appetite was showing signs of returning. The only concrete remnant of the treatments was the tattooed dots.

I suffered some very serious gynecological side effects from the radiation. Luckily, Cindy had been on top of things, warning me in advance that I would suffer a lot of physical damage. Neither she, Dr. Menzel nor Dr. Silberstein knew to what extent that would manifest. After my surgery, my gynecologist would offer me several options for treatments to make sure my sex life would survive the radiation side effects.

At the start of chemotherapy, I was told that the drugs would most likely cause infertility, killing off that last ovary. I wanted no more kids, anyway. That ovary was marinated in chemo for 12 weeks and deep fried 29 times by radiation. All the doctors reassured me I was no longer fertile. Technically, there was nothing to talk about where this was concerned, yet it was always on my mind.

Considering the confidence of my doctors, my obsession with having that one remaining ovary removed was inexplicable. It was all I could think about. I decided to talk to Dr. Quilici about it during my upcoming surgical consultation. I would not leave his office without his capitulation. Thankfully, I did not have to resort to begging. He agreed to remove it during the reversal surgery, much to my relief. I was looking forward to losing my colostomy, but I was even more excited to be ovary free.

As for the rest of the contents of my abdomen, Dr. Menzel reassured me that the radiation damage to my internal organs was purely physical injury and that there were no physiological changes. With time, the damage would heal and repair. Again, patience was the prescription.

I worried about how difficult it was to gain weight after radiation. The scale was stuck on one number, no matter what I ate or how many calories I consumed. None of my doctors seemed concerned, and every time I brought it up, they told me to stop obsessing over it. I was missing a large stretch of my colon; my digestion was changed. Preparing for the upcoming surgery would make me lose a couple more pounds. And then the recovery would make it difficult to eat enough to gain them back. It could be months after surgery before I saw the scale creep upward again. Each one of them said, "This is just what you weigh now." My nutritionist pointed out that my body was in full-time recovery mode, using all its resources to repair and rebuild the injured organs inside me by eating up every calorie I ingested. It was not interested in storing fat yet. She told me to enjoy this period of my life when I could eat anything I wanted and not gain a single ounce.

Inflammation affected every tissue. IMRT spared nothing. The nurses and technicians were correct: my ability to regulate my body temperature was completely gone and would not return for many weeks. I could be chilled one moment and then burning up the next. I needed to sleep with the windows open at night. In those cooler autumn months, Louis shivered next to me under his extra layer of blankets while I was covered in a layer of sweat.

I wanted to hike, but the soaring temperatures of an autumn heatwave were prohibitive. So, I spent my afternoons on the sofa binge-watching *Star Trek: The Next Generation* interspersed with episodes of *90-Day Fiancé*. I ate potato chips, handfuls of nuts, and sugar-free chocolates while alternating between hot flashes and icy chills. Each morning, I hit the yoga mat, but carefully replaced precious calories after each practice, hoping to bank extra fat on my deflated butt cheeks.

My body had reached a point of exhaustion from the continual onslaught of drugs and radiation and decided it needed a break. My body had learned to survive on the fat stores in my hips, breasts, and butt cheeks. I was flat all over. Now, my body was pulling the metaphorical covers over its head and refusing to entertain visitors.

Amanda was right: watching my hair grow back was one of the greatest affirmations of recovery. It was amazing how unsettling the difference in color (Luna and I had the same graphite hair color now), texture (it was baby soft), and volume (it was thick and wavy) were to me. My expectation was that as my hair returned, I would see a return to my familiar reflection in the mirror. So, it seemed petulant that I was annoyed at the healthy hair growth. It was unruly, unshaped, and wild like Muppet fur. I was so self-conscious of how bad it looked. Despite everyone's reassurances it looked fine and not to worry, I covered it up. I wore headbands and barrettes because wearing a scarf or a skullcap to hide it felt too much like chemo. I no longer wanted to look like a cancer patient, but I still wanted the world to know about my accomplishment. What I really needed was a T-shirt that read, "Nice Try Cancer."

I was beside myself with excitement when my hair was so out of control that I needed to schedule an appointment with my hairstylist, Amy, who I had not seen since before this all began. I spent the days leading up to the long-anticipated coiffing imagining an impossible transformation. When I arrived at the salon, she greeted me with an enveloping hug, lifting me off the ground, and squeezing me as close to her as possible. I missed her so much that it was hard not to break down into tears right there in front of the other clients. She cleaned up my messy hair and made it a bit more feminine. Her professional bird's-eye view from above discovered that my part had moved to the other side of my head. When she got through with me, I no longer looked like a little Sasquatch. I looked like a put-together woman with an incredible story to tell.

Nothing like a best friend to put things into perspective. Lori responded to the *after* photo: "Of all the ridiculous shit cancer has asked of you, now you have to change the direction your hair parts?!" Two thousand miles between us, we roared with laughter over the airwaves. "Let me know when you become left-handed!"

My hair was just the outward sign of my recovery, proof that the drugs were losing their grip on me. I was looking in the mirror and seeing a dark shape in the static gradually coming into focus. I learned to laugh again without breaking down into tears. I felt what it was like to take a deep breath and exhale without screaming. I was able to joke with Ria at the cancer center who conducts the COVID screening: "Do you have any COVID symptoms today?" And to answer with my favorite response, "Nope, just the cancer!"

It was also about being able to drive myself to appointments, singing along with The Cure while flying across the valley like a newly licensed teenager. I went close to seven months without driving, so getting behind the wheel was a major milestone. Not so many months earlier, it seemed likely that I would not see my upcoming birthday. Now here I was, two months past my expiration date, on the 118 Freeway, amused, dare I say delighted, by the congested traffic at the 405 interchange.

An unexpected thing happened during this period: I missed Dr. Jacobs and everyone in his office. It was a strange sensation, very much like missing my school friends during summer break. I was seeing them every two weeks for my routine blood work. But in between, I had a dull ache in my heart for them. As my next appointment on the calendar creeped closer, I became giddy. I even started having dreams about everyone. I suppose forming an attachment to the people who saved my life was unavoidable. It was astounding just how much I loved them.

These were the people that saw me at my worst and could make me feel normal. They steadied me when I had dizzy spells and cheered when I gained a single pound. When I cried in the middle of a perfectly normal sentence, they never flinched; they reassured me that everything I was feeling was normal. They treated my colostomy like another medical reality, took cues from me when I made *dad jokes* about it, and laughed at Louis when he asked if there was an elective surgery to cure me of those.

·   ·   ·   ·   ·

I was feeling better than I had in over a year; my energy levels were pretty high despite how easily I got out of breath with the slightest exertion. A few more late effects of both treatments began appearing. Radiation had left me with a clunky limp because of the scar tissue that had formed within my pelvis, and for some inexplicable reason, my shoulders dramatically cracked and popped. Thanks to chemo, my eyes were dry and scratchy, which made it impossible to wear my contact lenses. Turns out that my prescription had increased, which was why I was squinting through my 1-year-old progressive lenses. I had lost so much weight that my wedding rings were loose, and I was worried they would fly off if I made any exuberant hand gestures.

My brain took its sweet time rising out of the chemo fog. Suzy and I met for lunch at an outdoor cafe without masks, the first time we had actually seen each other's entire faces. More than once, one of us would start a sentence and then trail off. "What in the world was I saying?" And we would both break out in gut-busting laughter, since neither one of us could remember what we had been talking about.

I found it difficult to allow myself to indulge in the hope that there was not any significant cancer left inside my body. Alice reminded me once again that "Someone riddled with cancer doesn't have the amount of energy you do." She was right. Just a year ago, I had experienced the energy drain of an undiscovered parasitic cancer. Just as there had been no mistaking that something was the matter with me, there could be no mistaking that I was on the mend.

At my radiation follow-up, one month after my last treatment, Cindy handed me some light reading entitled *Healthy Living After Cancer*. There had not yet been a scan, test, or exam saying that I was cancer-free. Yet, there she was, handing me the resource packet. I read every single word on every single page. I read the information about the other cancers, the ones that I did not have. She had given this to me, on that particular day, because she saw something I was struggling to accept: obvious well-being. Five days later, I would get confirmation that things were heading in the right direction.

No matter how much I worried, or how many sleepless hours I spent, nothing would change the outcome of the PET/CT the next morning. Louis and the dogs snored peacefully while I tossed and turned. At 3 a.m., I kicked off the blankets, wondering if I should just get up and watch tv in the living room. I was uncertain if the surge of energy I was feeling was hopefulness of a clear scan, or fear that this scan would reveal something more horrible hiding in my pelvis. I avoided allowing my exposed foot to dangle over the edge of the bed, the old childhood bogeyman fears alive and well, the same way I was avoiding allowing my mind to dangle over that deep dark chasm where bright hope lurked.

On August 22, 2022, I lay inside the machine for my third PET/CT scan in 9 months. Both doctors, Jacobs and Menzel, had already told me they expected nothing to show up on the scan, and I desperately wanted to believe them. The machine slowly pulled me through, taking images of my insides while I envisioned healthy organs and positivity flowing through me.

Unlike my previous scans, I would not have to wait several weeks, or even days, to get these results. Just two hours later, the email notification arrived that the results had been posted to my medical portal. I took a deep breath, signed in, and began reading the scan out loud to Louis. As expected, the head, neck, chest, and skeletal scans were normal.

My eyes hesitated on the title of the next section, afraid to allow my gaze to drop to the first bullet point. My vision became tunneled, my mouth went dry, and I attempted to read the word jumble that declared my fate:

Abdomen and Pelvis:
1. Normal physiological activity within the kidneys, ureters, bladder, and gut
2. No mesenteric or pre-sacral PET avid adenopathy within the pelvis
3. No hypermetabolic asymmetry to indicate neoplasm in this current study

Impression :
1. Negative PET/CT fusion scan
2. No abnormal neoplastic activity

At first, I could barely speak the words. Then I could not get out of the word loop: no abnormal neoplastic activity. Negative scan. No adenopathy... no abnormal neoplastic activity. Negative scan. Negative.

Negative.

The familiar tears started flowing. The build-up of stress, fear, anxiety, anticipation, disbelief, and hope gushed out of me all at once. I could hardly breathe. Is this possible? Did I just beat Stage-4C colon cancer?

No. I could not possibly be this lucky. But was it luck? Or had the very real, focused attention, expertise, and goodwill of an entire team of people, coupled with my moxie, made this happen? Luck played no part in this. My exhausted body and exhausted husband were a testament to that.

I alone tolerated four surgeries. I alone endured 12 weeks of chemotherapy. I alone suffered through 29 rounds of radiation. I alone lived in my head where the scary monsters hung from the rafters like giant bats waiting to swoop down and snatch me away. Louis' hand and voice were often the only things that kept me tethered to this world.

Later that afternoon, as I sent screen captures of the PET results to my family, I quickly noted that I was not sharing in their enthusiasm and excitement. Though everyone around me was cheering for the good news, I was feeling skeptical at best and cynical at worst. My parents celebrated on the phone, and I was becoming more apathetic. Credulity had turned into ambivalence. I was not just rejecting the news; I was pushing back against everyone's joy and zealously trying to ruin it for them.

I spoke with Ella later that afternoon. "I'm having a hard time staying excited about this news." It was harder to accept there might not be any more cancer than it was to accept the cancer in the first place. She reassured me that the range of emotions we experience is vast, and not to put pressure on myself to feel a certain way.

Suzy's words played in my head: "I don't think I can take this news at face value." It was hard to accept that my overall condition was improving and that the end of the road could be a few weeks away on Dr. Quilici's operating table. I just had to get there. I should be enjoying the good news and expecting no extra stresses ahead of me. Instead, I was snapping at Louis, breaking into tears for no apparent reason, not answering texts or phone calls, and pushing everyone away from me so I did not have to face the good news.

I had a scary surgery coming up and there was no way around it. I would have to tell the whole world what was happening. Now I was stressing about how much I would share in my blog. Would I come right out and report, "I had a clear PET scan, and everyone expects this to be the end of it." Or would I play the role of press secretary and toe the party line: "This is just an exploratory surgery." I decided I was not even going to bring up the colostomy reversal this time; I could not bear the thought of going through that again in public. Besides, how much goodwill and excitement did I want to have directed at me?

The truth was, I just wanted to be left alone.

I decided not to tell anyone else about the supposed clear PET results. And I especially did not want to tell Suzy the details. She had asked for an update on my scan, and although I answered her right away with a generic answer, several days passed without a response from her. I never thought that she might be upset with me. I just had a bad feeling. Because I did not have her husband's phone number, there was no way to find out what was going on. She was five doses into her second round of chemo, and although that is pretty badass of her to endure 11 total treatments so far, I was certain that something had gone wrong.

When she eventually got in touch with me, it was confirmed that she was not doing as well as me. I felt it was more important than ever to not talk too much about my situation. I had to give her the support she needed now. After an acute attack of severe abdominal pain, they sent her for an emergency CT scan. A new lesion had appeared on her liver despite the 11 rounds of chemo she had already endured. No one would know what it was until another PET/CT, scheduled for three weeks from now. As the end of chemo neared, she expressed the same feelings I had experienced between treatments. There is relief in knowing chemo is over, yet deep terror at spending the next few weeks with no treatments.

I could at least take a breath knowing that she was alright for now. Even with this latest setback, she sounded like herself: positive, strong, and brave. I would not feel better until I saw her with my own eyes. During this stretch of time, our visits to the cancer center had not coincided, and I was craving her company. I started making plans to sit with her during her sixth infusion.

"There is no justice in this world." Dr. Kagan's words played over and over in my head. I felt guilty for doing so well while Suzy was encountering setbacks. My chemo was seemingly successful with one round, six treatments. And here she was, going through a second round with no clue if it was working. I wondered often if she resented me, even though she said many times that she was happy for me, and also glad that she would avoid radiation treatments after watching what I went through.

I was moody and emotional and could not properly articulate what I was feeling. Of course, Louis wanted to talk about it. I tried to explain how I felt but was no closer to naming the most mysterious feelings than I was before. He is deeply empathic. He desperately wanted to grasp what I was saying, yet I felt like I was explaining an alien world to him with such a glorious landscape that the only adjectives were tears. Although I felt strong and physically ready for this upcoming surgery, I was tired of fighting cancer.

To add to the emotional storm, I realized I was mourning the end of the journey. Was it possible? Was I upset that there may not be any more treatments on the horizon? Was I hoping for more drugs or radiation? Was I hoping that Dr. Jacobs would tell me there was still some cancer left to fight? Why was I clinging to cancer like a security blanket?

I could not imagine a life without the weekly trips to the cancer center, without a fistful of pills every day, and without side effects to soothe. How was I supposed to live without *The Abdominable:* my monstrous pet? I no longer knew how to not be a cancer patient anymore. Without ongoing treatments, how was I ever going to stay well? I could think of all the things in the privacy of my head, but once I said them out loud, the truth of it would become real.

I was *afraid* of being healthy.

I wanted to get on with the surgery, but the thought of the final preparatory steps was exhausting. I did not want to make the appointment for my pre-op physical; I did not want another nasal swab for COVID; and I absolutely did not want another nurse making life span predictions while they prepped me for major surgery. I dreaded the thought of more hospital food, stumbling to the bathroom with the IV tree in the middle of the night, and doing tedious laps of the ward. And then I would think, *but Suzy has another chemo treatment,* and perspective would come rushing back.

It was impossible to avoid the way I was feeling. I was tired of being special. I was tired of the millions of texts and emails. I was tired of asking Louis to help me around the house. I was tired of thinking about cancer. I was tired of driving to Burbank. I was tired of having to eat to gain weight. I was tired of everyone looking at me like I might break. I was tired of not working. I was tired of everyone telling me how cute my new hair was. I was tired of living in a fishbowl.

I was tired of being tired.

. . . . .

Life slowly returned to normal as I got back to my usual routines. *Normal* could mean anything I wanted it to now. It could even mean living without cancer casting a shadow over everything I did. I started to be able to spend multiple minutes without thinking about cancer, or treatments, or worrying about what might be festering inside me. When I woke up during the night, I could turn my mind toward the mundane things like bills to pay or emails to send and listening for Andrew as he returned late at night. I did not need to panic about what the cancer might be doing inside of me.

Certain personality quirks were reappearing, like my general ambivalence toward eating, chronic insomnia, and combative morning attitude. As I tried to fall asleep each night, my legs buzzed with electricity, my feet tingled, and I tossed and turned. I had bursts of energy during the day that allowed me to exercise and tackle a few menial household chores. I spent the afternoons writing on the patio or practicing my cello.

My body was healing from the assaults it had endured from chemotherapy and radiation. Black skin was flaking off from the burns; the skin on my hands was softening. Since contacts were out of the question for a while, I splurged on some fun blue glasses. *Hey, I survived cancer! I deserved to be a little quirky now.*

Six weeks after radiation, everyone saw I was getting back to my usual self. Dr. Jacobs noticed the improvements at my pre-op check-up, saying he could see my recovery just by looking at me. He did not know me before cancer, so he never experienced how nimble my conversation skills are. I have to work hard not to interrupt people if they do not speak fast enough for me. But not Dr. Jacobs. His conversational pacing meant we were both vying for airtime. The entire office witnessed my true rhythms, making it more clear in retrospect just how much chemo and radiation had knocked me down.

I had to adjust to the subtle changes in my physical body. This made yoga almost as difficult as it was when I first started learning to do it. The tendons, ligaments, joints, and muscles of my pelvic structure were taking a long time to heal. Until the cancer had struck, I had enjoyed very flexible hips. I was one of those people that could easily put their legs behind their head. But now, that movement was restricted thanks to the new scar tissue. Simple forward folds to grab my toes became a struggle, as tightness and discomfort screamed through the backs of my legs. The simplest poses were agony, and my outright frustration was difficult to mask even while all alone in the privacy of my yoga-slash-music room.

I would have to accept the changes in my body, because they may not turn out to be temporary. Embracing my new body would be an important part of moving forward with my emotional healing. The more I railed against my tight hips, the tighter they became. It would be easy to work through the physical effects, compared to the Herculean effort it would take to fix the mental effects. Where would I find the emotional strength I needed to get through this?

On the yoga mat one morning, my body fighting every single pose I was throwing at it, something popped in my hip and my head. In that instant, I felt my attitude change from frustration to compassion. This body, which I was trying to push to do yoga the way it used to, was no longer the same. It had survived a deadly disease that consumed a couple of organs; it bounced back from multiple surgeries with blinding speed; it had been poisoned by systemwide chemotherapy; it was bombarded with radiation and burnt to a crisp. After each of these assaults, my body recovered. It did some amazing things, not the least of which was saving itself from cancer. Yet here I was, frustrated that my foot was not going behind my head.

I broke down into tears when I finally understood just how ridiculous I was being. *Ungrateful* was the word that flashed through my brain. It was true. I was being ungrateful for the amazing gifts this little body had given me in these 10 months. These were shameful tears, which once they ran their course, turned penitent. From this point on, I would be thankful for the new body I had. I would wear all the scars on my belly as a badge of honor. I would remember to hug myself now and then.

This is a body that survived.

WELCOME TO THE BRIGHT

The morning of my first surgery, December 9, 2021, had been dark and stormy, uncharacteristic conditions for Southern California. We had laid together, entwined in my hospital bed, while waiting for the nurses to collect me. Louis was unsettled and anxious as I was being wheeled away, convinced that no good news was about to come back to him. He had nothing to hope for that day other than that I might survive the surgery. Sitting in my room, waiting for the surgeon to find him with the update, as unlikely as it sounds, he watched a rainbow form over the mountains across the valley. It gave him a tiny glimmer of hope. He held on to this image throughout all 10 months of my treatment.

On Thursday, September 22, 2022, 42 weeks later, we were quiet as we dressed and prepared for what I secretly believed would be my last surgery. This autumn morning was the exact opposite. Pleasantly warm, sunny, and clear, we discovered peace, allowing ourselves to give in a little to that ever-elusive hope. We could hope there was no cancer. We could hope I would not have too much pain, and we could hope I might come home sooner than five days. For the first time since this all began, we could even allow ourselves to hope I might come out of this perfectly healthy. Whatever we dared to dream, we could dream it in the bright blue sunshine.

The morning was filled with many signs that this would be a good day. A serenade of a nearby coyote chorus awakened us just before dawn. We were amused when my hawk friend took up in a tree in our backyard to scream at the morning songbirds, Louis commenting on how alike that hawk and I were in the mornings. I explained to Dusty and Luna that I would be home in two wake-ups, allowing myself to hope that I would come home early. We even arrived at the hospital 15 minutes early thanks to the unusually clear traffic.

This time, my pre-op nurse was infectiously positive, keenly interested in my story, and most importantly, not making survival predictions. Even though I had not told her my exact issues, as soon as she found out that I had radiation, she waxed poetic about a gynecological oncologist who could treat the stricture. It was the same doctor that Dr. Kagan had recommended at the start of this story: the one that we did not see. This time, we were not screwing around. I vowed to make that appointment as soon as I got out of the hospital.

They gave Louis and me a private moment to say our goodbyes before they wheeled me off to the operating room. The bowel prep the night before had been tiring. The cleanse is similar to a colonoscopy but with the addition of three rapid doses of heavy antibiotics. Unlike the previous surgery in May when I was given the antibiotics in pill form, this time the hospital pharmacy had given them to me as suspensions. I was frustrated: I had made it through all that chemotherapy and radiation without a single retch, yet those bitter and gooey antibiotics almost brought me down. All of that felt like something that had happened to me a year ago. It was so distant in my head as they pushed me down the now familiar hall toward the operating rooms.

The gurney could not move fast enough. I was looking forward to sliding onto the table. As they rolled me into the operating room, I heard a familiar song playing while the nurses prepared the room for me. *Journey* was blasting from the stereo: "Don't stop believin'!" The nostalgic vocals tickled a happy place inside me.

Right then I knew everything would be ok. I told the nurses that this was my brother's favorite band. The anesthesiologist administered the first sedatives. "It's definitely a good sign!" one nurse said, bright eyes shining over her mask.

I was feeling so giddy, and now a little dizzy. I broke into song myself. "Don't stop believin'!" I sang into the oxygen mask the anesthesiologist had placed over my mouth and nose.

The two nurses on either side of me sang along as they stretched out my arms and undressed me. Their voices reached me through the fog as the drugs washed over me and removed me from the present tense. I wonder how long I continued to sing after my memory cut out. Louis joked he was certain I put on quite a show for them, and they probably had trouble getting me to shut up long enough to get the breathing tube down my throat.

The next thing I knew, the music had ended, but the scenery was the same. They had awakened me in the operating room, helping me avoid the disorientation and panic that I had experienced in the past when waking in the recovery area. I was not up to speaking yet. I had more important matters to attend to: I needed to feel if the colostomy was still there.

My hand felt a flat bandage. *Don't stop believin'...* Shush. I was not ready to believe it. I tucked my arm against my side. I would wait for the drugs to wear off a little more before attempting another feel. By the time we returned to the recovery area, I was ready.

The colostomy was gone.

The sharp pain in my abdomen quickly dissolved in a flood of morphine. Now, I could focus on my excitement. If the colostomy was gone, did that mean good news where the cancer was concerned? I did not want to think too much about it yet. I was determined to stay calm until I saw Dr. Jacobs or Dr. Quilici. *Just don't stop believin', Lisa. You've come so far.*

Since I was already awake, my stay in recovery only lasted a few minutes. Before I knew it, I was being whisked back to the seventh floor, where familiar nurses tended to me and got me settled in my room. "We'll have you up and walking later tonight," the nurse stated matter-of-factly. She handed me a cup of cherry ice, which I dove into without hesitation. *Tonight?* I could hardly imagine that, but if I learned anything over the last 10 months, it was to never underestimate my body.

I knew that Dr. Jacobs always began his morning rounds at 5 a.m. I would only have to wait a few brief hours before I would hear *some news.* What that news would be, I did not have the time to speculate; I had things to do. I needed to get up in a couple of hours to walk (I did three laps at 11 p.m., just eight hours post-op) and I needed to sleep (I did not sleep). What I did not need was to run far-fetched scenarios in my head all night long.

I was already awake at 5 a.m. when an excited knock heralded Dr. Jacobs' arrival. "The surgical notes are posted!" He rushed to my bedside and took my hand in his. "I wanted to be the one to tell you: no sign of disease."

I just stared up at him. "What?" He had not spoken a single word of discernible English. Without Louis there to translate, I had no hope of understanding him.

"No disease," he repeated, slower and louder this time for us non-native speakers.

I do not know how long it took for me to take my next breath because it felt as if time had stopped. My ears filled with pulsing blood. I squinted up at him. "Is that for real?"

He laughed affectionately and patted my hand with his free hand. He said, "It's for real," in such a confident yet positive way that I knew it was permissible to believe him. I took his hand in both my hands and held on as tight as I could. I feared if I loosened my grip, he would float up and fly away. I wanted him and the good news to stay with me.

My tears flowed despite my paralysis. He was talking, though I did not hear what he said. I could see his jaw moving under his mask; I heard his voice break through the storm clouds a couple of times. "This is real," he repeated.

The week before my surgery, at my pre-op physical, Dr. Kagan had hugged me. "Do you know you are a miracle?" There was no way I could have understood his statement before I saw Dr. Jacob's reaction. I had the rest of my life to reconcile my good fortune against the incomprehensible odds that everyone had mercifully kept from me.

Later that morning, when Dr. Quilici arrived to repeat the news, I felt sober and intellectually ready to hear it again. "Surgery went well. Your colostomy is reversed. Ovary removed. And no visible disease present," he said, in what had become my favorite speaking voice of this cast of characters.

"You know, you saved my life." He tried to wave me off in his usual airy way, but this time I interrupted. "No, no, no, you have to accept my gratitude for this. If you hadn't acted so fast in December, I don't think I'd be here right now. You did save my life. So... thank you."

He may not be used to people manhandling him into listening like that, so I do not take it lightly that I somehow softened him into a mere mortal. "You beat the odds." And before he left the room, he squeezed my foot through the blanket. "You did good, young lady."

•　　•　　•　　•　　•

A short 48 hours after surgery, I was doing so well that Dr. Quilici said I could go home. I was positively giddy with excitement. I was farting without tearing my newly connected colon to pieces and gobbling up everything on my hospital tray. Having walked 30 laps of the ward before 11 a.m., I was about as energetic as someone could be so soon after major abdominal surgery.

Before changing into my street clothes, I asked nurse Lizette to bring me some cleansing wipes, convinced I smelled like a feral cat. Louis helped me with my impromptu sponge bath. I glimpsed my naked body in the mirror and felt a rush of affection at the sight of the bruises and bones. A little thinner than I remembered, I would soon find out when I arrived home that I had come close, but thankfully had not reached the mythical 20-pound cancer weight loss milestone. I had lost some ground with my weight in the last couple of weeks, but I looked stronger than I ever had. All those muscles that had carried me through chemo and radiation were still there, loud and clear at the surface. These arms could deadlift my body out of the bed. These legs carried me around the ward faster than most of the other patients (*Hey, Lisa, this isn't a race!*). These abdominal muscles, though chopped to bits, had required no pain meds since surgery.

It was more than ok for me to take a step back and marvel at what I had accomplished. I stared at this incredible little body that had willingly, and unfalteringly, fulfilled its duty.

"I think I almost died," I said, breaking the silence. Louis tenderly wiped my arm, the weight of the last 10 months rising and falling with every breath.

"Yeah," he whispered back, suddenly laser-focused on cleaning my elbow. We continued on in silence.

My abdomen boasted a collection of latex bandages, Tegaderm, Dermabond, and sutures. I took count of how many scars I would have after this. Five across my lower abdomen. I guess the possibility of becoming a middle-aged bikini model was officially off the table. Dr. Quilici had reopened the six-inch vertical incision from the December surgery that ran from my pubic bone to just under my belly button; he had closed the stoma location with a two-inch diagonal incision; and added at least three more *poke* holes during the laparoscopic portion of the surgery.

I was full of air, my abdomen visibly distended. Whenever I moved, the free-floating air would shift and irritate my diaphragm, which caused my neck and shoulders to ache. When I did my laps the day before, the nurses had encouraged me, "The only way out is through. Don't shy away from the pain. Just keep moving."

I continued to chant that none of this would last forever. "This is all temporary," Dr. Jacobs' most important words echoed in my head continuously. I reminded myself that no matter how *real* it felt at this moment, in a few days, this would all be just another dissolving hummingbird in her nest.

After dressing and collecting my belongings, it was time to leave St Joseph's Hospital: the place where, over the last 10 months I experienced the entire spectrum of emotions, formed attachments to nurses, was charmed by middle-of-the-night screamers, and witnessed actual miracles. I would not go so far as to say I would miss the hospital, but the monolith stood as bookends to my story.

For ten months, my life had been consumed with fighting for my life. It would have been easy for me to be overwhelmed with resentment and anger over this experience. But walking to the elevators, the flashing memories of this period were only positive ones: Nurse Lou's gentle voice, Dr. Jacobs' hugs, sunlight in Suzy's hair, Dr. Kagan's kiss on my forehead, Abby's laugh, an orchestra feeding my family, and more joy than I have ever experienced before. I was never alone.

I was not going to ride out of the hospital in a wheelchair. I wanted to walk on my own power. Cancer had tried to take everything from me. It had stripped away pounds, internal organs, hair, and skin, but it would never strip me of my life.

I stepped out of the elevator into the hospital lobby. Despite my sore belly and slow pace, I was a diva making her grand entrance. "Ta-Dah!" This was not the end of the opera. This was just the introduction of the winged, phantasmagoric character after the Entr'acte. This is where things get real!

Ashley, the nurse who accompanied me on this grand excursion back to the outside world, reminded me that my dogs were waiting for me at home, and they would help me heal even faster. She spoke about anecdotal evidence suggesting that people with pets have better cancer survival rates. I realized how true that was for me: the pull of getting home to Dusty and Luna was overwhelming. It broke my heart to know that if I did not return, they would sit by the front door for the rest of their lives, waiting for me. I needed to get home. Drowning out that sad thought, our wake-up doggy cheer, "Hooray! Hooray! A brand-new day!" resonated in my head. I promised myself I would chant this mantra with the dogs every morning from now on. Every morning that I am lucky enough to open my eyes deserves a celebration.

We stepped through the front doors and onto the sidewalk. Louis had parked the Subaru in the queue, the cars lined up like some sort of after-school pick-up. After two days in the ward, the bright sun hit my eyes like daggers. I was a newborn baby abruptly thrust into the white light of the world.

Louis waved to us and called out, "Welcome to the Bright!" He rushed over to collect me. I knew he was talking about the sunlight, but at that moment, it seemed like an appropriate title for the second half of my life.

I had beaten the odds, accomplishing the impossible. And I had walked away from cancer the same way I had walked in: on my own two feet.

EPILOGUE

Even after the chase with my dogs, the rabbits continued to pop out of the garden to play in the open grass in the early hours of each morning. Surely, they knew the dogs could reappear at any moment to chase them again. I wanted to believe that the rabbits did not appreciate the danger stalking them. Innocent little creatures who were unaware that they were tempting fate.

But it was difficult to see them in this simplified way. I wanted to believe they sensed it was safe to play in the yard. Living in the present moment, they could see the yard was empty of danger. They were free to enjoy the grass, untroubled, in full view of the mortal danger locked behind the patio door. No matter how excited the dogs were to get out and chase them, the thin pane of glass and the gatekeeper with the flashlight represented safety and freedom.

The surgical pathology report told an unnerving story. The pathologist discovered an adenocarcinoma hidden deep within the extracted ovary. Called a Krukenberg tumor, this metastasis of the colon cancer to the ovary was not visible to the PET or Dr. Quilici during surgery.

"What compelled you to ask me to remove that ovary?" he asked during my post-op appointment one week later. "If you had not asked, I would have left it alone. It appeared to be a normal ovary."

Although I doubted he would believe my fantastic experience with dreams and visions, I still told him about my obsession and the need to have it out. I never ignore these kinds of persistent messages. "I just decided I had to ask you to do it."

"It may have been the best decision of your life." He indulged me in a rare hug to conclude our appointment.

The next day, Dr. Jacobs confirmed that although there were no visible signs of disease, I would begin taking two drugs, Xeloda and Avastin, as adjuvant treatment, "To hedge our bets." A recent bone scan revealed that osteoporosis had occurred — another side effect of chemotherapy. I would have to receive treatments for this new condition as well.

Going into this appointment, I had tried to imagine Dr. Jacobs saying, "You're cured! Carry on." No matter how hard I tried, it was impossible to imagine. In my heart, I knew that something else was coming, and I found comfort in the new treatment plan. Calm as he described the schedule for the next year, I felt an emotion a lot like relief washing over me. There was nothing scary about this next step. I was going to be eased back into my post-cancer life with training wheels.

Louis, on the other hand, was visibly punctured and taking on water. "I'm exhausted for you." I felt sorry for him as we sat together on the patio later that afternoon. He stared quietly toward the mountains in the distance beyond our yard. "I had really hoped that this was over."

Taking a handful of pills every day and driving to Burbank to get a 30-minute infusion every three weeks was the thin pane of glass between me and *The Abdominable*.

All I had to do was trust my doctors to keep the glass door between myself and cancer locked and under constant surveillance with their powerful flashlights. Then, just like the rabbits, I would be able to pop out of the garden bushes and enjoy an empty and safe yard.

It was time to play in the grass again.

COVER IMAGE

What do you see in the book's cover? Is it despair and sadness, or hope and bravery? What is the right emotion to feel, and to assume I am feeling when you look at that picture?

The truth is: this is just me practicing squats during a yoga class. I was not thinking anything in particular when I took the original photo except, "Please let this be the last squat." Otherwise, there is no deep emotion attached to this image.

When I published this photo on my blog, many people thought I was diving into a deep depression; they feared I might even be suicidal. I got a lot of texts "Are you ok?!" It was amazing how quickly people attached a negative perspective to a photo, especially a photo of someone with cancer.

I meant the photo to elicit powerful emotions from everyone who sees it. Let it serve as a reminder that projecting your own fears and perceptions onto a cancer patient might do more harm than you realize.

I see this photo as a yoga victory. Squatting is one of the more difficult poses for me. I see my heels flat on the mat and celebrate the year of hard work it took for me to be able to do that.

So, if you see this picture and think, "Poor Lisa is really suffering," think again. This photo shows me doing something very strong to ensure that I survived cancer.

This is a photo of Super Lisa

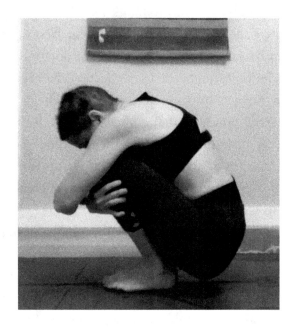

ACKNOWLEDGMENTS

The creation of this book, but more importantly, my survival, depended on some very important people:

There is no adequate way to thank *The Team of Grown Ups*: Doctors Lee Kagan, Phillipe Quilici, Edwin Jacobs, and Paul Menzel. The baton was handed off from one doctor to the other with grace, humility, and dare I say affection. Before this, I had never been hugged by a doctor, and through all of this, I experienced the power of that connection. Dr. Jacobs' report upon meeting me in the hospital for the first time opened with: "I entered the room to find a very pleasant woman lying comfortably." When I read this, I knew he was going to make sure that I would live.

They saved my life because they "crossed the streams," their collective intentions aimed straight at me, and the coming together of powerful energy to accomplish something unimaginable. I can find no way to thank them properly with words. They gave me the gift of the second half of my life: The Bright. The only sure way to thank them for it is to accept it with humility and then make something of it.

My husband, Louis Febre, was equal parts my foundational rock and tireless cheerleader. He was strong when I was weak, and he was honest when I needed lucidity. I told him that he had the harder job through all of this, and I still believe it. He held me when I cried for no reason and reassured me when I had a million reasons for the tears. He is my heart, my dearest partner, and my soulmate. In the randomness of this universe, we were reunited. Because of him and his strength and love, I came through this and emerged as my better self.

My son, Andrew Jenkins, showed me how tough and how vulnerable he really is. Throughout this experience, he was strong when I needed support, entertaining when I needed a laugh, and loving when I needed a son's love. He was the first person to hear the words "I'm so scared" come out of my mouth. He comforted me, and while he held me in his arms, I thought of all the times I held him as a child. As he stands on the edge of adulthood, I am so proud of who he is and who he will be. He is a treasure, and I am so lucky to be the one to call him my own.

Lori Stone has been my best friend since we were 12 years old. She was by my side, every step of the way, despite the miles. She was there to reassure me, more than once, that hummingbirds always build new nests. She was there to catch all the emotional pieces that flaked off of me at random times every single day. She always knew the exact right jokes to pop a stitch or two. She is and will always be more of a sister than a friend; and although there were thousands of miles between us, I could always feel her with me.

Pamela de Almeida, Ella Davies, and Alice Scherwin. I don't think there is an appropriate way to say thank you to these women. They wrapped me in their strength and wisdom, kindness and compassion, empathy, and ass-kicking. They could refocus my head when I could not see straight and gave me the permission I needed to freak out. They each protest when I say to them, "I couldn't have done this without you," but it is the truth. More than once, they let me sling an arm over their shoulders to be dragged back to the battlefield. All I can say is "Thank you" and hope that it is enough.

To Suzy Lee, my sister-in-arms. An instant love and a deep bond that can never be broken. Thank you for letting me into your world and for accepting my first tentative steps toward this friendship. Things aren't ever as scary when I know you're still here in this world. I don't know how you always found the strength to be there for me when you were suffering. I only hope I was able to give you even half of what you gave me. We will always be alone together in the garden, hiding, but never cowering, from The Abdominable.

To the doctors that worked in the background to support my diagnosis and treatment: Dr. John Kasher and Dr. Taaly Silberstein. Their decisive and sober decisions saved my life, and their unfaltering positivity saved my head. Their selflessness and humility put me on the right path toward healing, and for that, I am grateful.

Thank you to the nurses, technicians, and essential support team who administered my treatments:

All my love and deepest gratitude to everyone in Dr. Jacobs' office: Lori, Letitia, Lucy, Debbie, and all the rest whose names floated away in wisps of chemo clouds. To Alex for sharing and connecting, and to Brian for literally holding me up when I couldn't stand.

My deepest gratitude to the staff of the Infusion Department, without whose positivity and shining lights I couldn't have done this: Abby, Terry, and Trish who administered the drugs along with a healthy dose of love, Odalys who worked tirelessly to accommodate my schedule, the "Chip Lady" and all the other nurses and volunteers who came in and out of focus.

To the nurses on the 7th floor at St Joseph's who saw me through my surgeries and recoveries: Ashley, Lucia, Esther, Alexis, Sara, Lou, Noralyn, Michelle, Alexander, Trish, Lizette, and all the others whose names I can't remember thanks to the morphine; Jessica, the best pre-op nurse, and to Mabel in the ER.

Thank you to Dr. Kagan's assistants, Carina, Joanna, Sandy, and Cindy; and to Dr. Quilici's endearing Type-A assistants: Tiffany, Dr. Tovar, and Mariceia.

To all those in the Radiation Department who tolerated my poor attempts at radioactive humor: Cindy, Terri, Paulette, Ignacio, and Elaine.

Humble grace to my nurse-navigator Martha Likins, who is an expert at soothing panic; Remy Peters, my knowledgeable nutritionist; and Briana Gaudioso, at reception, who cheerfully counted down to my last treatment.

To those friends who offered cancer stories, both their own and their loved ones, with honesty, transparency, and levity. They were infinite wells of support and friendship, but also full of the down and dirty information about the parallel universe of cancer. They willingly gave me the uncensored versions of their own journeys and gave me compassionate reassurance when I needed gentle encouragement. Without them, I would have been more frightened, more anxious, and more alone. They were a lifeline, and I cannot thank them enough for their friendship and kindness.

To Jeremy Reynolds for giving me something important to ponder, while reminding me to always laugh harder and more often than I cried.

Jeff McKinney and the team at *Anna's Wish*. I drew inspiration and courage from his daughter Anna's story and legacy. Consider donating to this wonderful nonprofit. annaswish.org

To everyone at Black Rose Writing who took a chance on a new author, especially Reagan Rothe, Minna Rothe, Lianne Bennett; and Dave Seaburn, for encouraging me to submit my manuscript. To the beta readers and editors who didn't laugh and burn the manuscript.

Thank you to everyone whose presence during my journey made all the difference in the world. No matter how insignificant you may have thought your contribution was, always remember that a single kind word can represent a universe of love.

To my family: Melissa Brunsting, Adrian Febre, Benjamin Febre, Roberto Febre, Alejandra Febre, Daniele Febre, Lorraine & Richard Gilmore, Ana & Joel Guzman, Claudia Guzman, Carolina Guzman, Joanna & Larry Smolen, Melissa & Todd Smolen.

To the Moorpark Symphony Orchestra: all the Musicians and Board of Directors; Gail Amendt, Sharon Cooper, Chuck Fernandez, Lecy Fredo, Judy Garf, Sean Matthes, Barbara Poehls, Lynn Olson, and Phyllis & Gary Rautenberg. They say people with pets have better survival rates, and the MSO was the ultimate "pet." Thank you for loving me back.

To all my friends who listened, reached out, and stood by me through this whole misadventure: Satsuki Crozier, Rhondda Dayton, Jennifer Deirmendjian, Cary Einberger, Helena & Michael Gatt, Amy Hateley, Michael Hrycelak, Rachel Leshaw; Christine Barbas, Carole Bloom, Dave Bristol, Cindy Anne Broz, Gary & Vicky Claussen, Kate Cohen, Jennifer Formell, Beth Lano, Donna Lill, Jacqui Marx, Eleanor & Nicole McPherson, Michelle Milner, Declan & Barbara Morden,

Sherry Wall, Liz Watts, Randy Weinstein, Mara Wolfgang, and Amanda Zidow; Neil Baker, Yvonne deSousa, Michelle A. Dick, Janet Jayasekera, Barbara Luker, Melinda Wolf, Emily Wright, and to all the rest who I did not mention by name.

PHOTO ALBUM

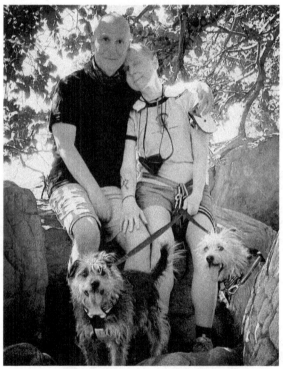

Taking a break while hiking during chemo, February 2022

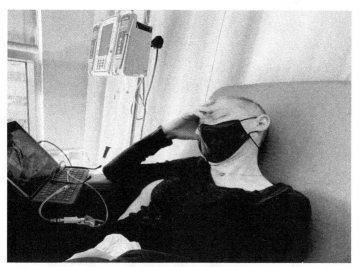

It's not all shiny Instagram posts
6th infusion, March 2022

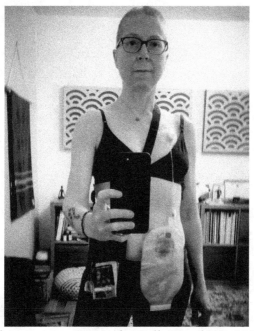

The morning I rang the Bell, March 18, 2022

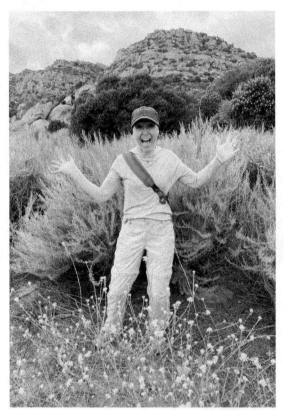

Hiking between chemo and radiation, May 2022

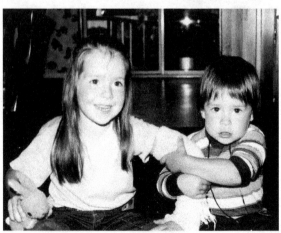

Lisa & Todd, 1978

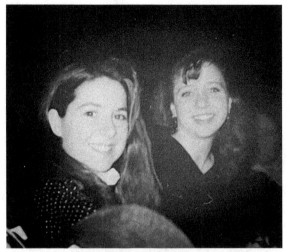

Lisa & Lori, 1992

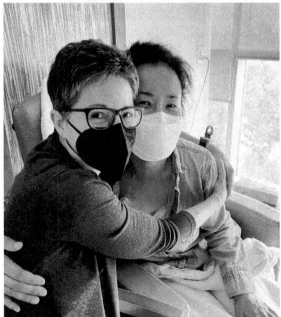

With Suzy during her last infusion

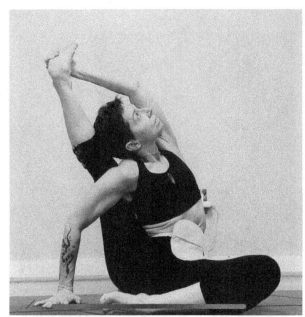

Yoga during radiation, colostomy and all!

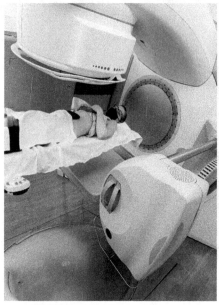

Radiation Treatment

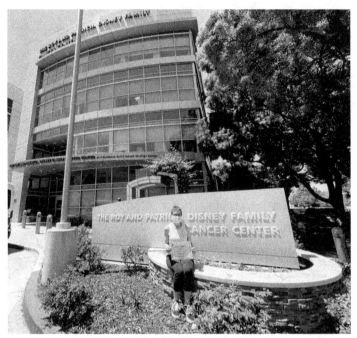

Last Day of Radiation, July 22, 2022

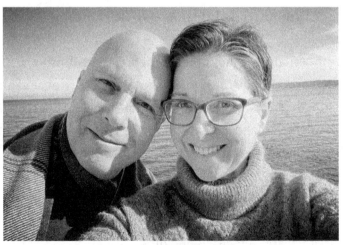

Living in "The Bright," December 2022

APPENDIX

Common Symptoms of Colon Cancer:

1. Unintended Weight Loss
2. Persistent diarrhea, loose stools with blood, rectal bleeding
3. Constipation with Persistent Pain
4. Loss of Appetite

It's now recommended that you get your first colonoscopy at age 45. No excuses: just go do it!!

Chemotherapy Infusion Day-Bag Packing List

Prescription drugs and other supportive medications, iPad, iPhone, earbuds, power chargers, book, snacks, ginger candies, light lunch, gloves, neck scarf, knit hat/headscarf, large water bottle (no ice), hand cream, lidocaine cream, hand sanitizer, wallet, ID and insurance cards. If you have a colostomy, remember your supply kit. Pack extra snacks or even a lunch for whoever is taking you to the infusion — it's likely they haven't thought ahead to what *they* might need during the day because they are so focused on you.

Radiation Day-Bag List

Prescription drugs and other supportive medications, a bottle of water, crackers or salty snacks, hand sanitizer, wallet, ID and insurance cards, ginger candies, and colostomy supply kit. Even though the visits are short, you will need medications and snacks with you.

How Best to Help A Friend During Chemo:

- Time your delivery of food and gifts to arrive in the 3 days leading up to their chemo treatment. During infusions, it is difficult to muster the energy to answer texts, and nearly impossible to face someone on our doorstep expecting to say, "Hello."
- Make sure all food gifts are frozen or tightly sealed and will last at least a week in the refrigerator. Often, we don't have an appetite during the infusion itself. We don't want to feel guilty knowing the food you put so much time and effort into is rotting in the fridge.
- Be sensitive to the types of foods your friend is eating during chemo. Food aversions are common, and although they can be difficult to accommodate, respect those limits. Remember, special diets like vegetarian/vegan, gluten-free, sugar free/diabetic, etc., still matter to your friend.
- Do not contact the patient while they are in the middle of chemo. Many infusions last multiple days; learn your friend's schedule. Feel free to send "Thinking of you" type texts, but don't send anything that requires a response, and don't call. Even something as simple as,

"Can I bring you anything?" can be monumentally overwhelming. Just hold off. When your friend emerges from their cocoon and starts responding to texts again will be a better time to ask, "What do you need for next time?"

- When you drop anything off, leave it on the front porch, and then move off to a safe distance. Text your friend, "Look on your porch!" either after you're in your car, or once you're driving away. It's not that the patient doesn't want to see you. It's that chemo damages our bone marrow, leaving us highly susceptible to infections.

- Surgical masks are a must if you are going to be anywhere near us, even outdoors. Hugs can be dangerous, so save those for celebrating the recovery! Just respect whatever limits the patient has regarding physical contact. It's not about you, it's about keeping them safe and healthy when they have low to no immunity.

- Offer to run errands. "Anything you need, just text me," is one of the greatest texts that I got. I never sent someone on an errand, but several people can attest to the fact that I broke down in tears on the phone every time this offer was made.

Supporting Your Friend

- If you or someone you love has had cancer and they belonged to a support group, please share that information with the newly diagnosed. They may or may not join a group, but just the knowledge that there are more people out there who went through the same type of cancer is comforting. I did not join a colon cancer-specific support group, but I joined a colostomy support group and the United Ostomy Association of America (UOAA).

- Any cancer, or long-term illness experiences you have to share, please do. Those who have beaten cancer give the best advice. Hearing from others who have recovered and are living normal lives is inspiring and necessary. It's a weird club to belong to, no one wants to welcome more people into it, but knowing my feelings and experiences were not unique went a long way toward my mental well-being.

- Offer to drive your friend to their treatments. Many people have 9-5 jobs and taking a day off to sit with a partner during infusions might be a problem in those situations. Offering to drive and accompany your friend to treatments, relieving the spouse of some of these duties, may mean the difference between high-stress and being able to breathe. If you know your friends are balancing work and treatment schedules, and you can do it, make this offer, and make it often.

Supplies and Gift Suggestions

- **Knitted Hats, Scarfs, Buffs** – My head got cold once my hair fell out. Since my scalp had never seen the light of day before, the hats also acted as sunscreen. Chemo makes everyone feel cold, so no matter the time of year, scarves, buffs, and hats are a must and there's no such thing as too many.

- **Soup and Soft Food** – The best thing to feed someone with a questionable appetite is a nutrient-dense soup. No chewing is necessary. Soft foods like hummus and homemade bread do wonders for the soul. Chewing can be treacherous when there are sores on your cheeks or tongue, so hard, sharp, salty, or crunchy foods can be difficult to handle. A friend of mine kept me fed with an endless supply of root vegetable purée soups that felt like a huge dose of nutritional love. Make soups that can be frozen and used when your friend needs them the most.

- **Gloves, Socks, and Slippers** – Cold sensitivity is a huge issue with platinum-based chemo drugs like Oxaliplatin. Light gloves, which allowed me to go about my daily business, were a perfect gift. Go crazy with the thickness of the socks you send and try to find slippers with hard or structured soles for walking stability. The cozier the better!

- **Skin Care** – Many chemotherapy drugs, as well as radiation treatments, cause severe skin reactions. Toss a few skin care treats into your gift basket, including: *Udderly Smooth* and *Miaderm*, CBD based skin creams, and calendula soaps. For ostomy reversal surgery recovery, use calendula diaper cream.

- **Food Delivery Gift Cards** – On days when the rest of the family is pacing around wondering what to do for dinner because mom is knocked down, those cards come in handy. It also means that you don't have to worry about the fresh meal you sent over going to waste. If you send a card, we can order whenever we want and when it's most needed.

- **Cozy Blanket** – During infusions, we tend to become chilled. Blankets are a great way to wrap us in your affection from afar. It's not just nice to have at the infusion center but is a comfort once we arrive home. My brother sent me a blanket that I carried around the house like Linus and even dragged out to the patio to sit in the sun with it wrapped around me.

- **Do Not Send Flowers** – As thoughtful a gift of flowers may seem, it's actually very dangerous for anyone going through chemo. At the very least, the intense scent of cut flowers can be very sickening to the patient. In my case, I had constant bloody noses and irritated sinuses made worse by the pollen. More to the point, cut flowers can bring microbes and tiny pests into the home. It can also exacerbate allergies and sinus infections. Instead of flowers, send a succulent, or choose something else from the list above.

HOW TO COPE WITH COMMON SIDE EFFECTS OF CHEMOTHERAPY (C) & RADIATION (R)

- <u>Fatigue (C, R)</u> – Rest. Don't over-exert yourself. Nap often, move slowly and allow your body this time to absorb the treatment unencumbered. The best way to regain some energy is to eat.
- <u>Cold Sensitivity (C)</u> – Wear light gloves and heavy socks at all times. Don't reach into the refrigerator or freezer. Warm any metal objects before you touch them barehanded. For mouth sensitivity, use children's, non-minty toothpaste and rinse with warm tap water. For the throat, only drink liquids that are warmer than room temperature. Take warm showers/baths and avoid cool swimming pools. *Never gulp, always take a small sip of everything first to test your throat's reaction.*
- <u>Hand/Foot Syndrome (C)</u> – The only cream that worked for me was *Udderly Smooth,* recommended by my oncologist. I would rub this into my hands, then put on light gloves. Do not pick at the peeling skin.
- <u>Burns (R)</u> – No matter where radiation is being applied to your body, you can count on some burns. I used a cream called *Miaderm,* which I applied twice a day and after every treatment. I also used calendula soap daily in the

shower. Once the burns appear, they won't heal until treatment is over. Continue to apply the cream, but once they turn into 2nd or 3rd-degree burns, you'll need a prescription burn cream from your doctor. With radiation treatments to the pelvis, you can expect burns between your buttocks and anywhere your skin rubs or reflects upon itself.

- Loss of Appetite (C, R) – Find easy-to-eat foods that don't challenge your taste buds. You may also lose your sense of taste, which could make it even more difficult to eat. Sometimes, sucking on a ginger candy before eating can wake up your surviving taste buds. Everyone is different, so once you figure out what foods you can tolerate, keep your kitchen pantry stocked. Even if you don't feel like eating, you should always try for some calories. There is a difference between loss of interest and loss of appetite. Many cancer patients crave spicy foods during treatment because that's all they can taste. If you aren't eating for more than 48 hours, contact your doctor.

- Weight Loss (C, R) – It's all too easy to lose weight with cancer treatments. No matter what, before any treatment begins, use the time beforehand to gain a significant amount of weight. My experience was that I needed between 5-8 pounds extra going into both chemotherapy and radiation in order to stay within an acceptable range. Make it your mission to maintain your weight within the range specified by your oncologist. Eat with impunity and abandon, these are medically necessary calories. If you are having trouble maintaining your weight, your doctor may refer you to a nutritionist for support.

- <u>Mouth Sores (C)</u> – Avoid foods that are too cold or too hot, as well as salty, jagged, crispy, or hard foods. Rinse your mouth several times each day with warm salt water. When brushing your teeth, use a soft or extra-soft manual toothbrush, children's non-minty toothpaste, and do not floss or scrape your tongue. Try to keep your mouth closed as much as possible to avoid irritating sores with your teeth.

- <u>Hair Loss (C, R)</u> – Keep your newly exposed head out of direct sunlight and cover it to keep yourself warm. It usually starts growing back within 3 months of your last chemo infusion. You will lose all your body hair during chemo, and within the area you're receiving radiation. Don't worry, it grows back!

- <u>Anxiety and/or Depression (C, R)</u> – Recognize the signs early and ask for help. Listen to others who observe a change in your behavior. Your oncologist may prescribe medications or refer you to a mental health professional. Talking to friends who are cancer survivors, or an organized support group, can make a big difference. Keep up with your exercise routine, keep in contact with your friends, and always try to live as normally as possible during treatment. Keep an open line of communication with your oncologist so that you always receive the help that you need during this most difficult time of your life.

MY SIDE EFFECTS OF FOLFIRINOX

This is the most comprehensive list of *my side effects* on FOLFIRINOX that I can provide. Everyone has a unique experience, so remember this list only refers to me.

Fatigue
Insomnia
Constipation
Diarrhea
Nausea
Hair Loss
Confusion, Chemo Brain
Difficulty Emptying Bladder
Anemia
Low White Blood Cell Count
Low Platelet Count
Intestinal Cramps
Swollen Eyelids
Gritty & dry Eyes
Flushed Face
Swollen Face
Bloody Noses
Swollen/Congested Sinuses
Dry and Peeling Lips

Mouth/Cheek Sores
Tongue Sores
Burnt Gums
Numb Mouth
Difficulty Speaking
Difficulty Swallowing
Acid Reflux/GERD
Loss of Taste
Loss of Smell
Loss of Appetite
Foul (metal) Taste
Cold Sensitivity in Hands, Feet & Mouth
Hand, Foot and Face Spasms
Loss of Fine Motor Control
Difficulty Walking
Pins & Needles in Fingers (neuropathy)
Shaking Hands
Hand/Foot Syndrome:
   Red, Burnt Hands
   Peeling Skin on Hands
   Swollen Hands and Feet
Fingernails Separating from Cuticles
White Lines on Fingernails
Joint Pain
Menopause

MY FOLFIRINOX REGIMEN

Chemotherapy Drugs (IV infusion):
Leucovorin Calcium (Folinic Acid)
5-Fluorouracil
Irinotecan
Oxaliplatin

Supportive Drugs (IV infusion):
Lactated Ringers – hydration
Atropine – antispasmodic to counter intestinal cramps
Fosaprepitant – anti-nausea
Ondansetron – anti-nausea
Dexamethasone – corticosteroid to relieve inflammation
Heparin Sodium – blood thinner

MY CANCER TIMELINE

<u>2021</u>
June – 7.6cm ovarian cyst discovered (right side)
August – Intermittent pain on the left side begins
September – Pain begins to dictate my activity level
October – UTI, swollen bowel, constant severe pain
November 1 – CT scan
November 17 – PET scan
December 7 – Failed colonoscopy
December 8 – Admitted to hospital ER
December 9 – Emergency Surgery: Sigmoidectomy, colostomy, salpingo oophorectomy, exploratory laparoscopy

<u>2022</u>
January 4 – Portacath installation, surgery
January 5 – First round of chemotherapy
March 16 – Last round of chemotherapy
May 5 – Exploratory surgery
June 9 – First radiation treatment
July 22 – Last radiation treatment
September 22 – Colostomy reversal (anastomosis), exploratory laparoscopy, salpingo oophorectomy. End of the book.
October 19 – Adjuvant chemotherapy began

THOUGHTS ON TWO
COMMON CANCER LABELS

I spent a lot of time grappling with the decision to use the label *Cancer Survivor* when referring to not just myself, but everyone in long-term remission within these pages. I know that this is one of those loaded words that people have mixed feelings about. We didn't choose to *survive* cancer any more than someone chooses to survive a plane crash. It brings with it some strong reactions from those who have been in my position.

In the end, I chose to use the label *Cancer Survivor* because it is accepted widely as a term that makes it clear, even to those who have not been touched by cancer, precisely who we are talking about: people who have been diagnosed and lived to tell the tale. Few people use the word *cured;* most prefer *remission.*

I used the term *Cancer Patient* to describe people actively going through cancer treatments and currently under medical care.

NOTE FROM LISA FEBRE

Word-of-mouth is crucial for any author to succeed. If you enjoyed *Round the Twist: Facing the Abdominable*, please leave a review online—anywhere you are able. Even if it's just a sentence or two. It would make all the difference and would be very much appreciated.

Thanks!
Lisa Febre

We hope you enjoyed reading this title from:

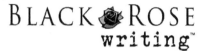

BLACK ROSE
writing™

www.blackrosewriting.com

Subscribe to our mailing list – *The Rosevine* – and receive **FREE** books, daily deals, and stay current with news about upcoming releases and our hottest authors.
Scan the QR code below to sign up.

Already a subscriber? Please accept a sincere thank you for being a fan of Black Rose Writing authors.

View other Black Rose Writing titles at
www.blackrosewriting.com/books and use promo code
PRINT to receive a **20% discount** when purchasing.

Printed in the USA
CPSIA information can be obtained
at www.ICGtesting.com
JSHW010705300823
47516JS00017B/307